FIRST FRCR ANATOMY
PRACTICE EXAMINATIONS

FIRST FRCR ANATOMY PRACTICE EXAMINATIONS

SHAUN QUIGLEY and SEAN FLANAGAN
Radiology trainees on the Barts and the London scheme

Edited by Dr Niall Power

Radcliffe Publishing
Oxford • New York

Radcliffe Publishing Ltd
18 Marcham Road
Abingdon
Oxon OX14 1AA
United Kingdom

www.radcliffepublishing.com
Electronic catalogue and worldwide online ordering facility.

British Library Cataloguing in Publication Data

A catalogue record for this book is available from the British Library.

ISBN-13: 978 1 84619 512 9

The paper used for the text pages of this book is FSC certified. FSC (The Forest Stewardship Council) is an international network to promote responsible management of the world's forests.

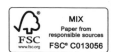

Typeset by Phoenix Photosetting, Chatham, Kent
Printed and bound by TJI Digital, Padstow, Cornwall

Contents

Foreword

The first year of radiology training can be a bewildering experience. New trainees, who have frequently occupied positions of authority and seniority on medical and surgical firms, must come to terms with their new status as radiology neophytes.

Among the wide range of new information to be learned perhaps the most important topic is radiological anatomy. Put simply, a thorough grasp of normal appearances on the full range of radiological modalities is essential if one is to learn the appearances of pathological processes to enable accurate reports to be constructed.

The Royal College of Radiologists, having abandoned the Part 1 exam featuring anatomy, physics and techniques several years ago, have recognised that reinstatement of a formal examination was required to ensure that radiological anatomy was learned thoroughly in the first year of training. The format chosen was of 20 images with five questions on each, usually of the 'name "A"' type, with occasional alternative factual questions to test knowledge further. This examination is now well established and in this book there are 10 practice exams of the identical format covering all body parts and imaging modalities.

Shaun Quigley and Sean Flanagan are, at the time of writing, 1st year radiology trainees in Barts and the London NHS trust and both passed the first sitting of the new exam in March 2010, upon which they immediately recognised that a book of practice exams would be of immense value to future candidates, and commenced the arduous task of collecting 200 images of all types, of exam standard, and setting five questions for each. They have accomplished this task very effectively and the result is a comprehensive, well structured and above all highly relevant book for all candidates approaching the new RCR anatomy exam.

I recommend this book highly to all such individuals.

Dr Niall Power
Consultant at Barts and the London
FRCR Part 1 Anatomy Module exam board member
June 2010

About the authors

Dr Shaun Quigley is a Radiology trainee on the Barts and the London scheme. After graduating from the University of Glasgow Medical School in 2006 he worked in Scotland and Sydney. His current interests involve squiring and Boris spotting. He is a jazz-funk aficionado.

Dr Sean Flanagan is a Radiology trainee on the Barts and the London scheme. Having graduated from Barts and the London Medical School he trained in Surgery with an interest in Orthopaedics before coming to his senses and moving to Radiology. He is a keen amateur cook and gourmand.

How to use this book

In the exam the candidate will be shown 20 images on a workstation with adjustable contrast but no other viewing aids. The answers are to be hand written on an answer sheet.

The mark scheme allocates two marks for each answer. Accuracy in identifying laterality is essential as where two marks are given for correct structure and side (e.g. Right Scaphoid Bone), only one mark is given for correct structure only (e.g. Scaphoid Bone). If the laterality is incorrect in your answer (despite a correct structure) no marks will be given.

Each of the 10 exams in this book also contains 20 images. A range of modalities are included, all of which are used regularly in clinical radiological practice. Each image depicts an area of normal anatomy and has five questions attached. The majority of these relate to the name of a labelled structure. In keeping with the format of the FRCR Part 1 Anatomy Exam however, we have included more detailed questions which test applied knowledge of the depicted anatomy.

To encourage a fair attempt at each question, we have elected to place the answers at the end of each exam.

The answers detail the imaging modality and study technique. We have also provided explanatory notes or study aids where relevant, and particularly in areas which often cause difficulties in clinical work.

For Isabelle, my family and friends and most of all,
my Mum to whom I owe so much
Shaun Quigley

To my parents for all they have done,
and Paula for putting up with me
Sean Flanagan

Exam 1

1.1

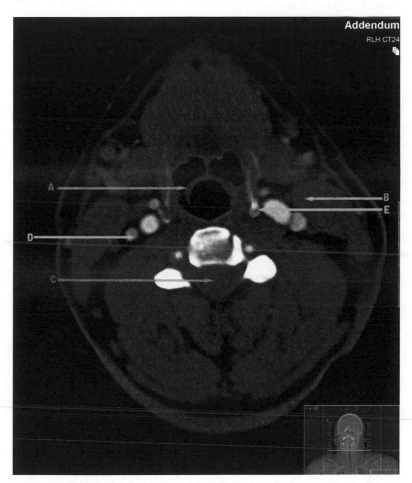

Answer the following questions.

1   Name structure 'A'.
2   Name structure 'B'.
3   Name structure 'C'.
4   Name structure 'D'.
5   Name structure 'E'.

1.2

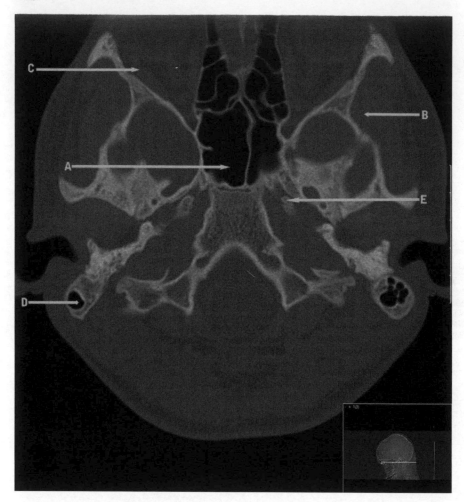

Answer the following questions.

1   Name structure 'A'.
2   Name structure 'B'.
3   Which cranial nerve supplies 'C'?
4   Name structure 'D'.
5   Name structure 'E'.

1.3

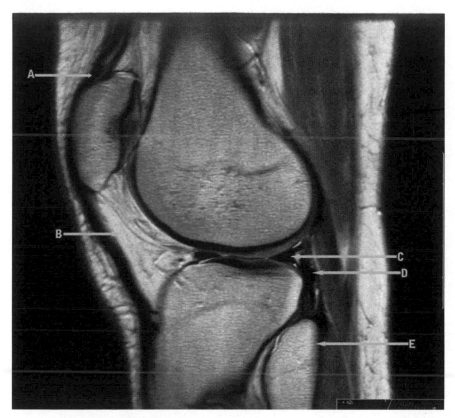

Answer the following questions.

1 Name structure 'A'.
2 Name structure 'B'.
3 Name structure 'C'.
4 Name structure 'D'.
5 Name structure 'E'.

1.4

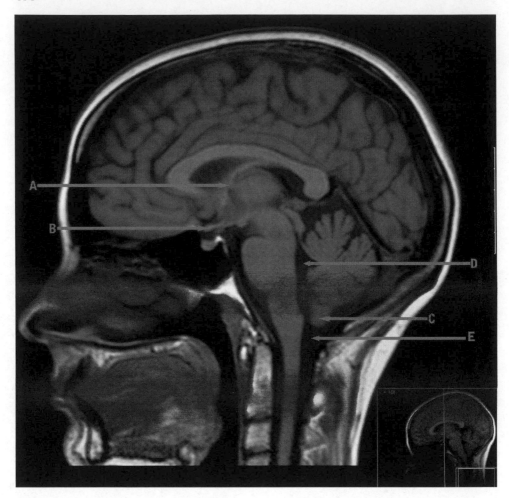

Answer the following questions.

1 Name structure 'A'.
2 In which CSF space is 'B' found?
3 Name structure 'C'.
4 What connects 'D' to the central canal of the spinal cord?
5 Which 3 structures link 'D' and 'E'?

1.5

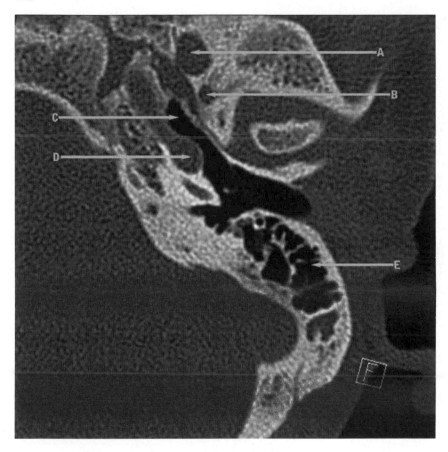

Answer the following questions.

1   Name structure 'A'.
2   Name structure 'B'.
3   Name structure 'C'.
4   Which structure passes through 'D'?
5   Name structure 'E'.

1.6

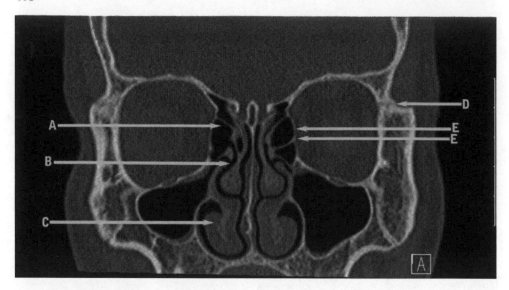

Answer the following questions.

1 Name structure 'A'.
2 Name structure 'B'.
3 Name structure 'C'.
4 Name structure 'D'.
5 Name structure 'E'.

1.7

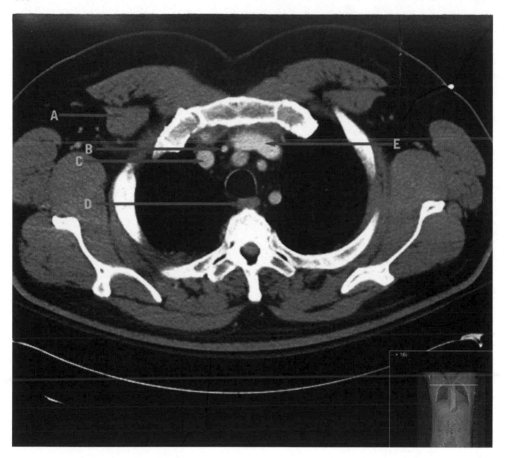

Answer the following questions.

1 Name structure 'A'.
2 Name structure 'B'.
3 Name structure 'C'.
4 At what vertebral level does 'D' pierce the diaphragm?
5 Name structure 'E'.

1.8

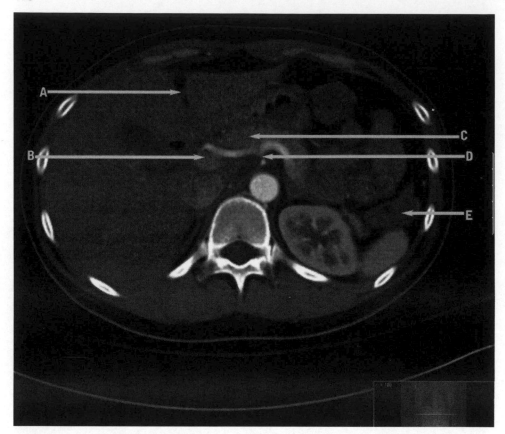

Answer the following questions.

1   Name structure 'A'.
2   Name structure 'B'.
3   Name structure 'C'.
4   Name structure 'D'.
5   Name structure 'E'.

1.9

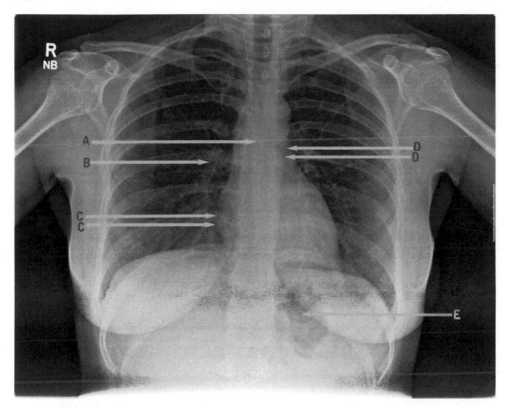

Answer the following questions.

1 Which cardiac chamber is found at 'A'?
2 Which two vessels form 'B'?
3 Which pulmonary lobe abuts 'C'?
4 Name structure 'D'.
5 Name structure 'E'.

1.10

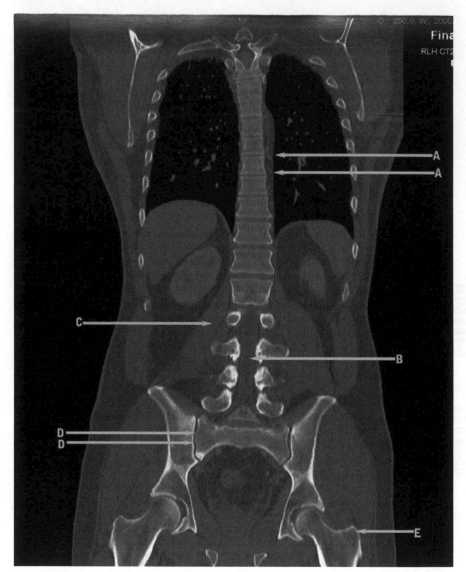

Answer the following questions.

1 At what vertebral level does 'A' pierce the diaphragm?
2 Name structure 'B'.
3 Name structure 'C'.
4 Name structure 'D'.
5 Name structure 'E'.

1.11

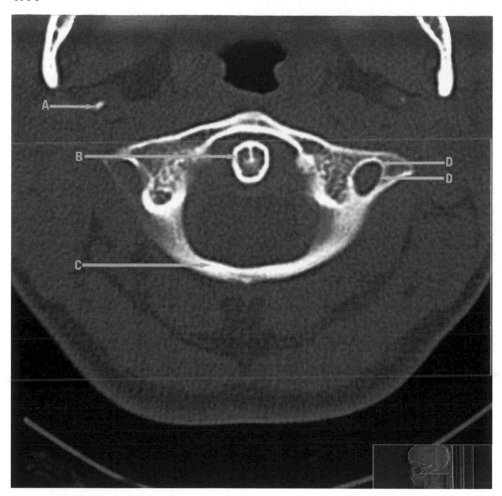

Answer the following questions.

1   Name structure 'A'.
2   Name structure 'B'.
3   Name structure 'C'.
4   Which structure passes through 'D'?
5   Which ligament attaches 'B' to the occiput?

1.12

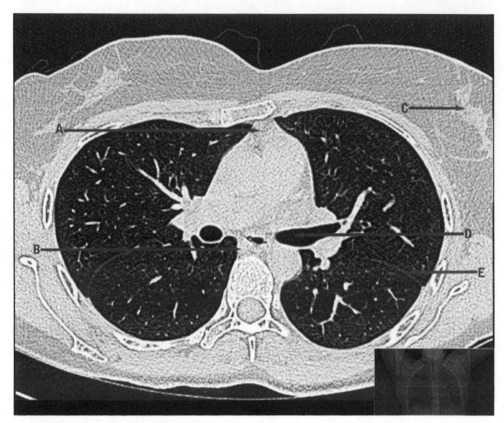

Answer the following questions.

1 Name structure 'A'.
2 Name structure 'B'.
3 Name structure 'C'.
4 Name structure 'D'.
5 Name structure 'E'.

1.13

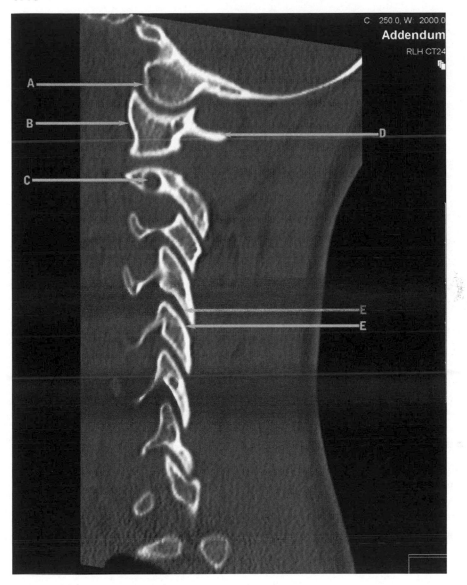

Answer the following questions.

1   Name structure 'A'.
2   Name structure 'B'.
3   Name structure 'C'.
4   Name structure 'D'.
5   Which ligament is found between 'E' and 'E'?

1.14

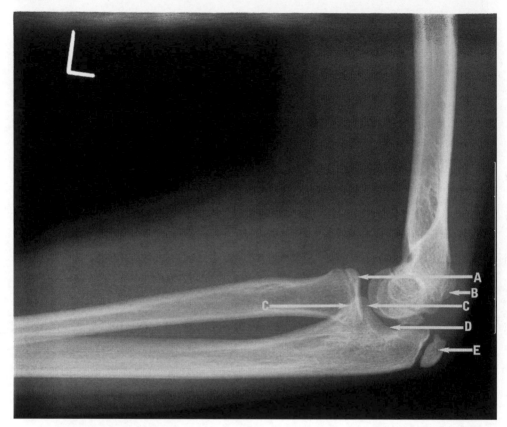

Answer the following questions.

1   Name structure 'A'.
2   Name structure 'B'.
3   Name structure 'C'.
4   Name structure 'D'.
5   Name structure 'E'.

1.15

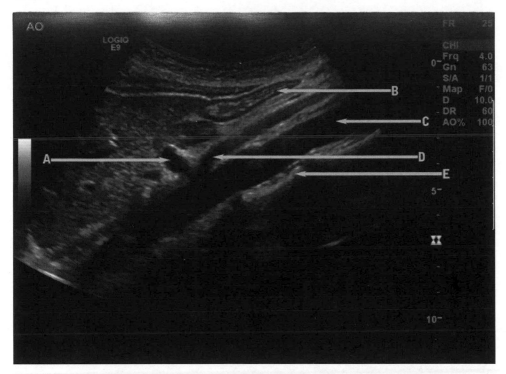

Answer the following questions.

1 Name structure 'A'.
2 Name structure 'B'.
3 Name structure 'C'.
4 Name structure 'D'.
5 Name structure 'E'.

1.16

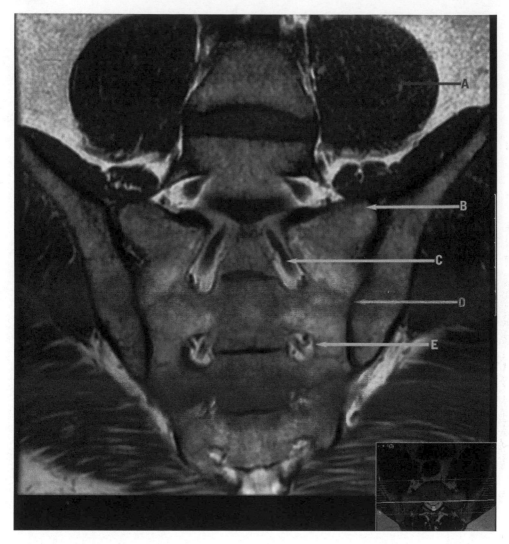

Answer the following questions.

1 Name structure 'A'.
2 Name structure 'B'.
3 Name structure 'C'.
4 Name structure 'D'.
5 Name structure 'E'.

1.17

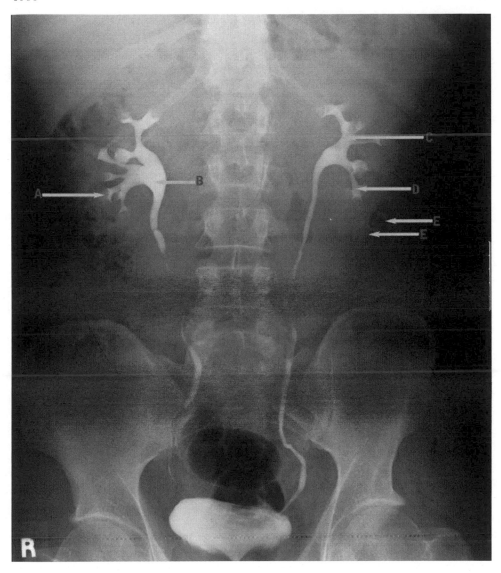

Answer the following questions.

1　Name structure 'A'.
2　Name structure 'B'.
3　Name structure 'C'.
4　Name structure 'D'.
5　Name structure 'E'.

1.18

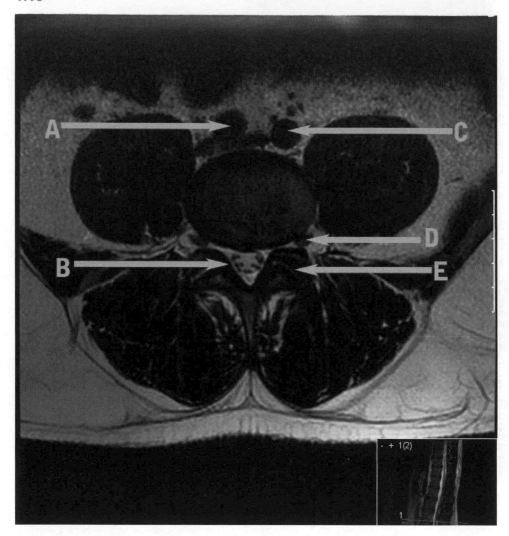

Answer the following questions.

1   Name structure 'A'.
2   Name structure 'B'.
3   Name structure 'C'.
4   Name structure 'D'.
5   Name structure 'E'.

1.19

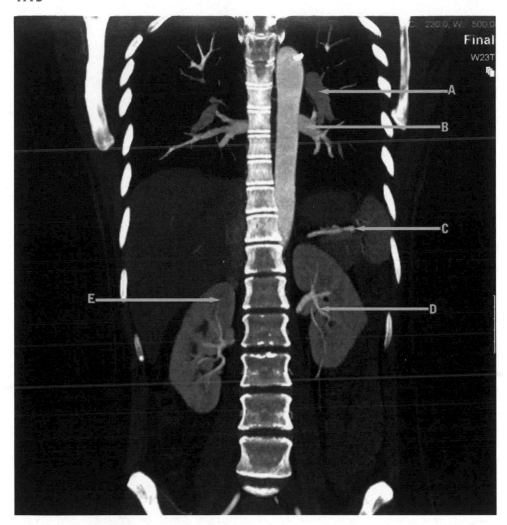

Answer the following questions.

1 Name structure 'A'.
2 Name structure 'B'.
3 Name structure 'C'.
4 Name structure 'D'.
5 Name structure 'E'.

1.20

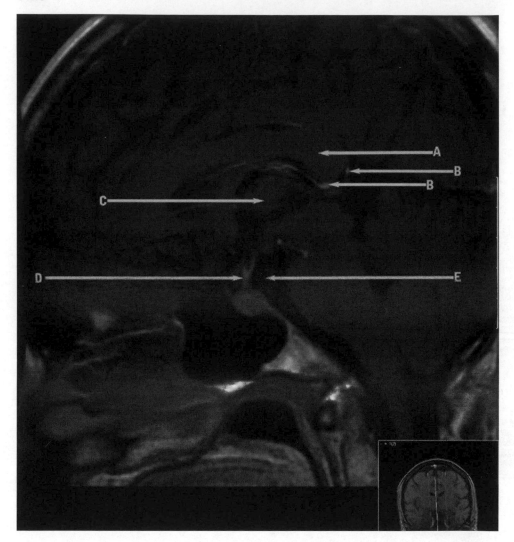

Answer the following questions.

1   Name structure 'A'.
2   Name structure 'B'.
3   Which artery supplies 'C'?
4   Name structure 'D'.
5   Name structure 'E'.

Answers

1.1
1   Right Lateral Glossoepiglottic Fold.
2   Left Sternocleidomastoid Muscle.
3   Thecal Sac.
4   Right Internal Jugular Vein.
5   Left Aspect of Thyroid Cartilage.

Axial contrast enhanced CT neck.

The window levels used have been chosen to maximise the information available on the vasculature – so-called 'angiogram' windows. This improved the contrast between the high attenuation vessels and the remainder of the neck structures. As a result, some differentiation between the various soft tissues is lost. The vertebral arteries are visible rising in the neck adjacent to the cervical vertebral bodies.

1.2
1   Sphenoid Sinus.
2   Left Temporalis Muscle.
3   Right CN VI.
4   **Right Mastoid Air Cells.**
5   **Left Petrous Apex.**

Axial CT base of skull – bone windows.

The carotid canal, through which passes the petrous internal carotid artery (ICA), is part of the temporal bone.

The greater wing of sphenoid is seen anteriorly. The lesser wing is located superior to this.

1.3
1   Quadriceps Tendon.
2   Hoffa's Fat Pad (Infrapatellar Fat Pad).
3   Posterior Horn of the Lateral Meniscus.
4   Popliteus Tendon.
5   Head of Fibula.

Sagittal MRI knee.

The menisci of the knee are fibrocartilage structures and appear low signal on MRI. Degeneration and tearing of these leads to oedema and therefore high signal within the structure.

Two ligaments attach to the posterior horn of the lateral meniscus (PHLM) – the meniscofemoral ligaments – these run from the PHLM to the lateral aspect of the medial femoral condyle. Named for their relation to the posterior cruciate ligament

(PCL), the anterior is known as the ligament of Humphrey, the posterior as the ligament of Wrisberg.

1.4

1   Fornix.
2   Suprasellar Cistern.
3   Cerebellar Tonsil.
4   Obex.
5   The Foramina of Luschka and the Foramen of Magendie.

Sagittal T1W MRI brain.

The paired foramina of Luschka and the midline foramen of Magendie allow CSF to flow from the ventricular system into the subarachnoid space at the cisterna magna. Obstruction to passage of CSF at this point will lead to dilatation of the lateral, 3rd and 4th ventricles. CSF also flows from the 4th ventricle to the obex and then through the central canal of the spinal cord.

1.5

1   Left Foramen Ovale.
2   Left Foramen Spinosum.
3   Left Eustachian Tube.
4   Left Internal Carotid Artery.
5   Left Mastoid Air Cells.

Axial CT temporal bone.

Convention indicates this is the left temporal bone.

The tensor tympani muscle is visible lateral to the Eustachian tube.

1.6

1   Right Anterior Ethmoid Air Cells.
2   Right Hiatus Semilunaris.
3   Right Inferior Nasal Turbinate.
4   Left Frontozygomatic Suture.
5   Left Lamina Papyracea.

Coronal CT paranasal sinuses.

The osteomeatal unit (OMU) is visible. Anatomical variation or pathology at this site impairs drainage of the maxillary antrum and can lead to sinusitis.

1.7

1   Right Pectoralis Minor Muscle.
2   Right Vertebral Artery.
3   Right Brachiocephalic Vein.
4   T10.
5   Left Brachiocephalic Vein.

Axial contrast enhanced CT chest.

1.8

1   **Falciform Ligament of Liver.**
2   **Portal Vein.**
3   Head of Pancreas.
4   Coeliac Axis.
5   Descending Colon.

Axial contrast enhanced CT abdomen.

Fat planes are of great importance in CT. The thin plane of perinephric fat separating the left kidney from the descending colon demonstrates the importance of recognising them – disruption of this plane in cases of renal cell carcinoma results in significant upstaging of disease.

1.9

1   Left Atrium.
2   Right Basal Pulmonary Artery and Right Upper Lobe Pulmonary Vein.
3   Right Middle Lobe.
4   Descending Aorta.
5   Stomach.

Frontal chest radiograph.

The visible vertebral bodies and azygooesophageal line indicate this is a 'high kV' radiograph. At high kV there is a reduction in radiographic contrast, reducing the contrast between soft tissue structures in the lung. This can make the diagnosis of parenchymal lesions more difficult.

1.10

1   T12.
2   Thecal Sac.
3   Right Psoas Muscle.
4   Right Sacroiliac Joint.
5   Greater Trochanter of Left Femur.

Coronal CT abdomen and pelvis – bone windows.

1.11

1   Right Styloid Process.
2   Odontoid Peg of C2.
3   Posterior Arch of C1.
4   Left Vertebral Artery.
5   Alar Ligament.

Axial CT cervical spine – bone windows.

The alar ligaments connect the lateral borders of the odontoid peg to the occipital condyles.

The dens is also attached to the clivus by the apical ligament.

The cruciform ligament serves to fix the dens to the anterior arch of C1.

1.12
1 Anterior Mediastinum.
2 Azygos Vein.
3 Glandular Tissue of Left Breast.
4 Left Main Bronchus.
5 Oblique Fissure of Left Lung.

Axial HRCT Chest.

The anterior mediastinum may give rise to pathology and in normal individuals should be composed of fat and therefore be of fat attenuation with a value of approximately –100 Hounsfield units (HU).

1.13
1 Occipital Condyle.
2 Lateral Mass of C1.
3 Foramen Transversarium of C2.
4 Lamina of C1.
5 Ligamentum Flavum.

Sagittal CT cervical spine – bone windows.

Widening of the space between the facet joints as viewed on sagittal images such as this can indicate severe traumatic neck injury. Absence of bony injury does not exclude potentially severe ligamentous injury.

1.14
1 **Centre for Left Radial Head**.
2 Centre for Left Medial Epicondyle.
3 Coronoid Process of Left Ulna.
4 Trochlear Notch of Left Ulna.
5 Centre for Olecranon of Ulna.

Lateral paediatric elbow radiograph.

The sequence of appearance of the ossification centres in the elbow can be memorised using the following mnemonic. This order serves as a guide only and variations do occur.

> **CRITOL**
> **C**apitulum
> **R**adial Head
> **I**nternal (Medial) Epicondyle
> **T**rochlea
> **O**lecranon
> **L**ateral Epicondyle.

1.15
1 Coeliac Axis.
2 Stomach.

3   Abdominal Aorta.
4   Superior Mesenteric Artery.
5   Vertebral Body.

Longitudinal US abdomen.

In thin subjects the aorta and vertebral bodies can be easily visualised. The abdominal aorta should be inspected during routine abdominal sonography in the elderly to exclude aneurysm formation. Paraaortic and coeliac axis lymphadenopathy can be identified by obtaining images at this level.

1.16
1   Left Psoas Muscle.
2   Left Sacral Ala.
3   Exiting Left Sacral Nerve Root.
4   Left Sacroiliac Joint.
5   Left Sacral Foramen.

Coronal MRI lumbosacral spine.

1.17
1   Renal Papilla of Right Lower Pole.
2   Right Renal Pelvis.
3   Major Calyx of Left Upper Pole.
4   Minor Calyx of Left Lower Pole.
5   Left Lower Pole of Kidney.

Intravenous urogram (IVU) – excretory phase.

This image is obtained approximately 10 minutes post injection of IV contrast. A CT urogram (CT IVU) performed at the same interval would produce axial images of the collecting systems and ureters. The CT IVU has replaced the conventional IVU in many centres.

1.18
1   Inferior Vena Cava.
2   Ligamentum Flavum.
3   Abdominal Aorta.
4   Exiting Left Sided Nerve Root.
5   Left Sided Facet Joint.

Axial MRI lumbar spine.

The cauda equina within the thecal sac is seen, indicating that this image is obtained below the level of the conus medullaris. The conus medullaris, the termination of the spinal cord proper, occurs at L1/2.

Facet joint degeneration is associated with ligamentum flavum hypertrophy. This can cause relative stenosis of the spinal canal and lead to radicular pain from impingement of exiting nerve roots.

1.19
1   Left Basal Pulmonary Artery.
2   Left Pulmonary Vein.
3   Splenic Artery.
4   Lobar Artery of Left Kidney.
5   Arcuate Artery of Right Upper Pole.

Coronal CT angiogram abdominal aorta.

The branches of the renal artery vessels can be appreciated. In patients who have undergone renal transplant, identification of these vessels using Doppler ultrasound is extremely important.

The arcuate vessels, seen towards the periphery, are used to measure the resistive index (RI) – a measure of resistance to flow within the renal vascular bed. The RI is a function of the peak systolic velocity and lowest diastolic velocity in the arcuate artery. It should be measured at several locations within the transplant and ideally should be less than 0.8. Higher RIs may indicate transplant dysfunction.

1.20
1   Splenium of Corpus Callosum.
2   Internal Cerebral Vein.
3   Posterior Cerebral Artery.
4   Pituitary Infundibulum.
5   Suprasellar Cistern.

Sagittal contrast enhanced T1W MRI pituitary gland.

The whole pituitary gland is seen as hyperintense. The nasal mucosa also appears high signal, indicating this is a post contrast image. MRI images acquired post gadolinium are T1W. Gadolinium shortens the T1 relaxation time of tissues, increasing the signal they return. High signal due to contrast is also visible in the internal cerebral veins.

Exam 2

2.1

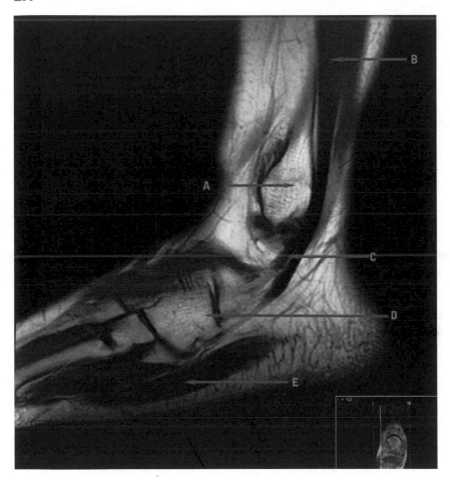

Answer the following questions.

1 Name structure 'A'.
2 Name structure 'B'.
3 Name structure 'C'.
4 Name structure 'D'.
5 Name structure 'E'.

2.2

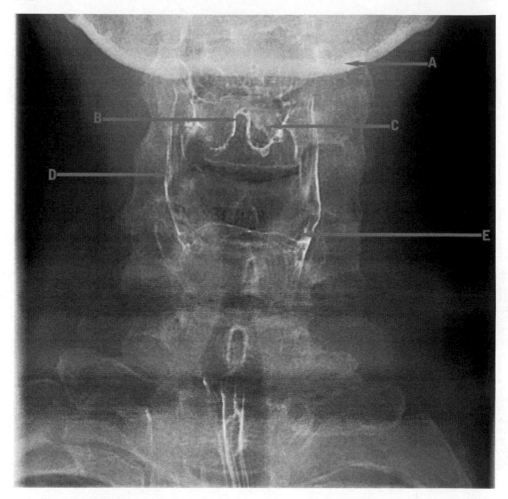

Answer the following questions.

1   Name structure 'A'.
2   Name structure 'B'.
3   Name structure 'C'.
4   What forms the wall of structure 'D'?
5   Name structure 'E'.

2.3

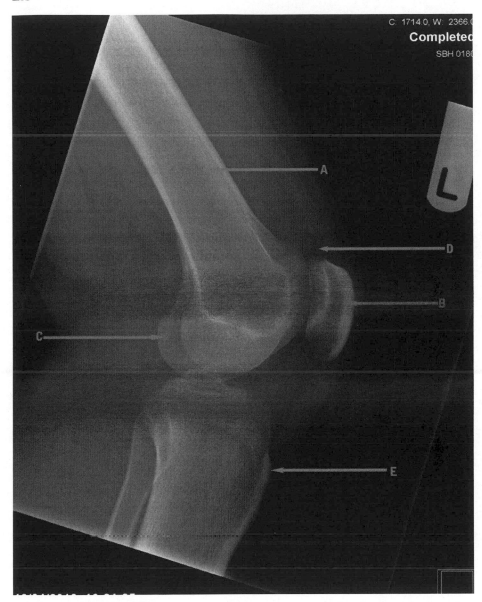

Answer the following questions.

1 Name structure 'A'.
2 Name structure 'B'.
3 Name structure 'C'.
4 Name structure 'D'.
5 Which structure inserts at 'E'?

2.4

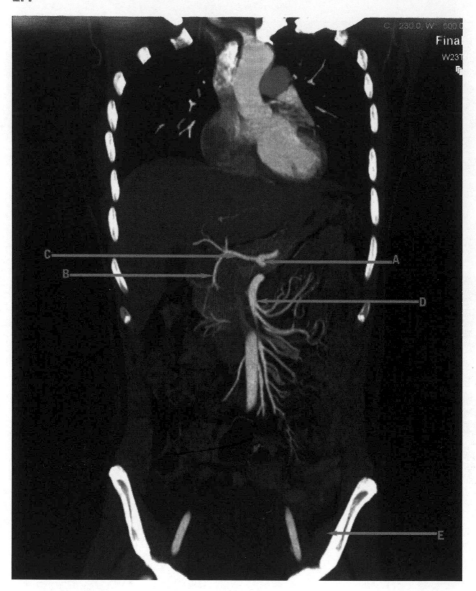

Answer the following questions.

1 At what vertebral level does structure 'A' arise?
2 Name structure 'B'.
3 Name structure 'C'.
4 Name structure 'D'.
5 Name structure 'E'.

2.5

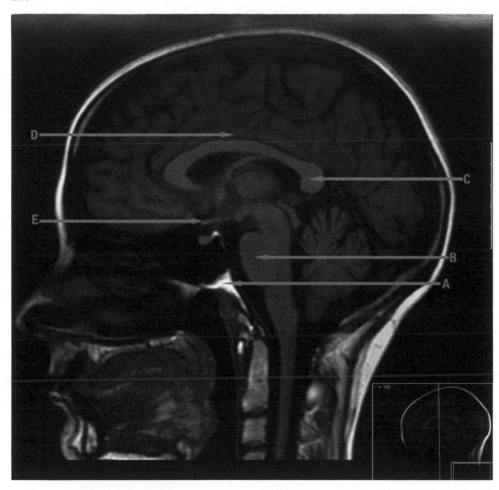

Answer the following questions.

1 Name structure 'A'.
2 Name structure 'B'.
3 Name structure 'C'.
4 Name structure 'D'.
5 Name structure 'E'.

2.6

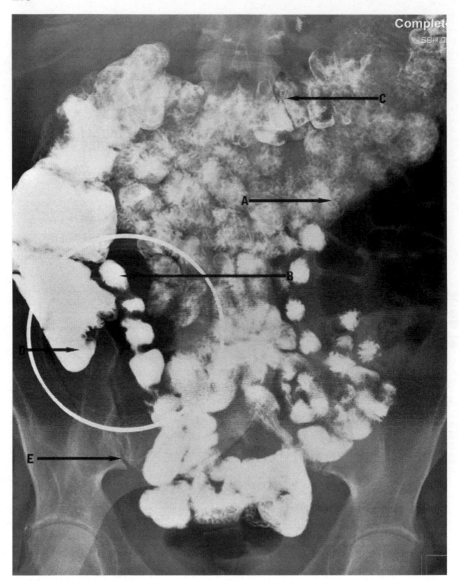

Answer the following questions.

1 Name structure 'A'.
2 Name structure 'B'.
3 Name structure 'C'.
4 Name structure 'D'.
5 Name structure 'E'.

2.7

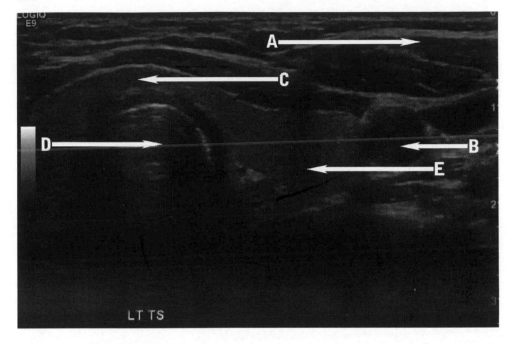

Answer the following questions.

1 **Name structure 'A'.**
2 **Name structure 'B'.**
3 Name structure 'C'.
4 Name structure 'D'.
5 Name structure 'E'.

2.8

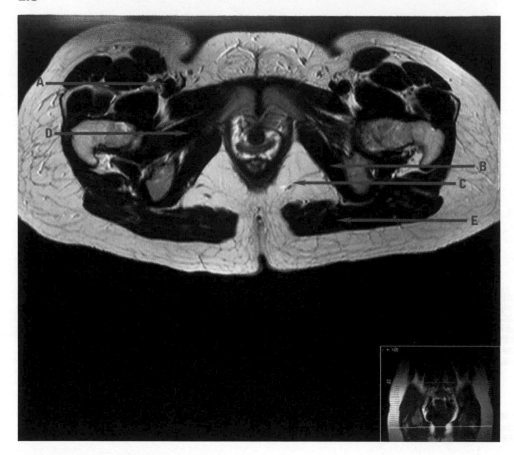

Answer the following questions.

1   Name structure 'A'.
2   Name structure 'B'.
3   Name structure 'C'.
4   Name structure 'D'.
5   Name structure 'E'.

2.9

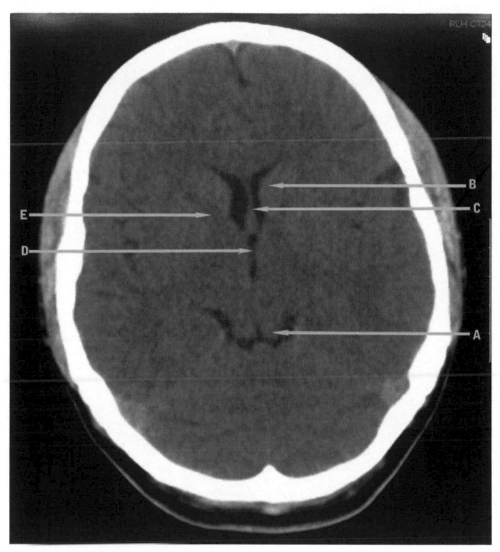

Answer the following questions.

1 Name structure 'A'.
2 Name structure 'B'.
3 Name structure 'C'.
4 Name structure 'D'.
5 Name structure 'E'.

2.10

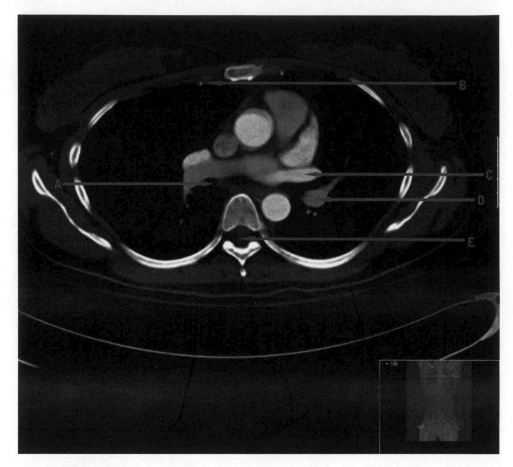

Answer the following questions.

1 Name structure 'A'.
2 Name structure 'B'.
3 Name structure 'C'.
4 Name structure 'D'.
5 Name structure 'E'.

2.11

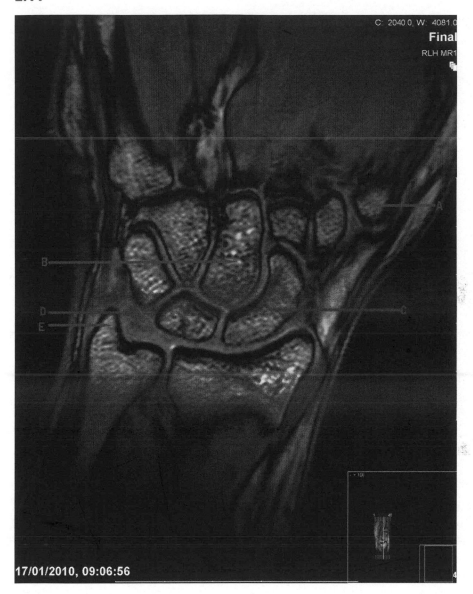

Answer the following questions.

1   Name structure 'A'.
2   Name structure 'B'.
3   Name structure 'C'.
4   Name structure 'D'.
5   Name structure 'E'.

2.12

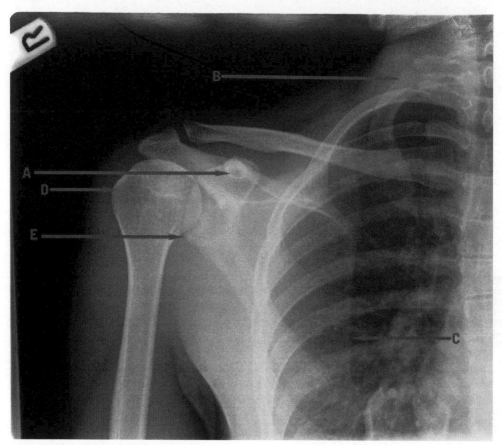

Answer the following questions.

1   Name structure 'A'.
2   Name structure 'B'.
3   Name structure 'C'.
4   Name structure 'D'.
5   Name structure 'E'.

2.13

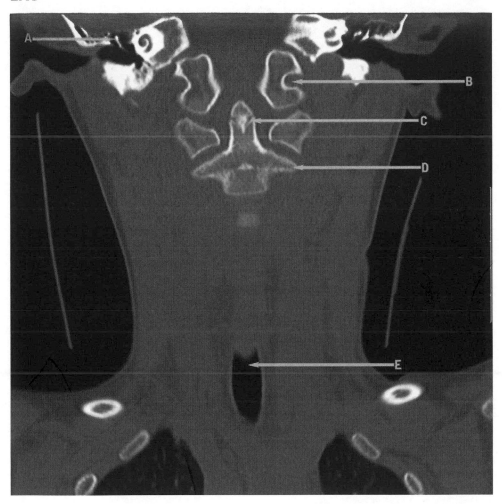

Answer the following questions.

1 Name structure 'A'.
2 Which structure passes through 'B'?
3 Name the anatomical variant 'C'.
4 Name structure 'D'.
5 Name structure 'E'.

2.14

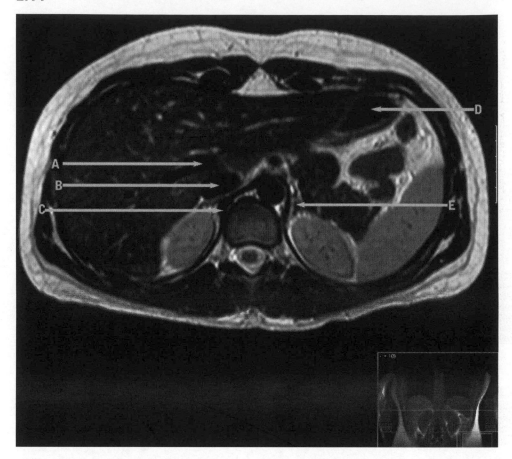

Answer the following questions.

1   Which structures form 'A'?
2   Name structure 'B'.
3   Name structure 'C'.
4   Name structure 'D'.
5   Name structure 'E'.

2.15

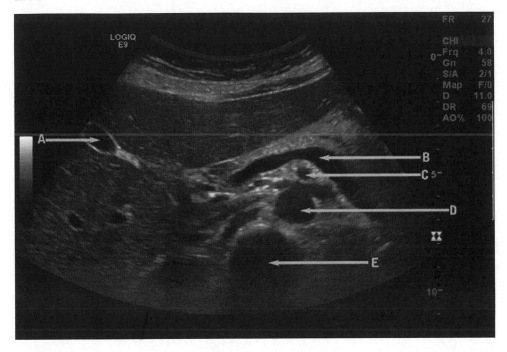

Answer the following questions.

1 **Name structure** 'A'.
2 Name structure 'B'.
3 Name structure 'C'.
4 Name structure 'D'.
5 Name structure 'E'.

2.16

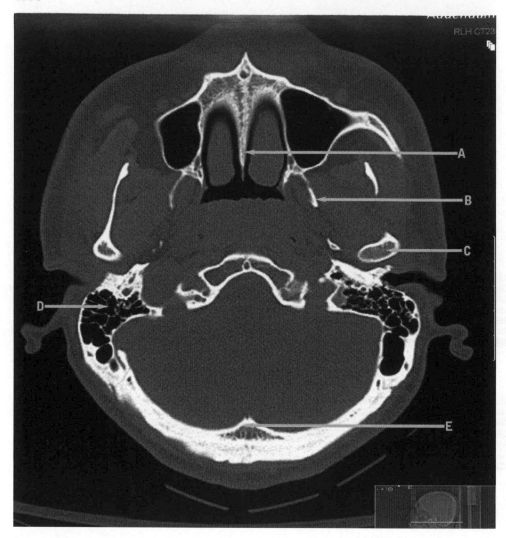

Answer the following questions.

1 Name structure 'A'.
2 Name structure 'B'.
3 Name structure 'C'.
4 Name structure 'D'.
5 Name structure 'E'.

2.17

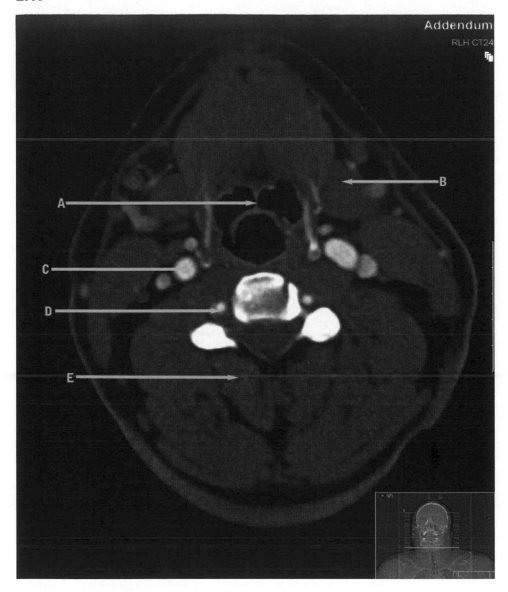

Answer the following questions.

1   Name structure 'A'.
2   Name structure 'B'.
3   Name structure 'C'.
4   Name structure 'D'.
5   Name structure 'E'.

2.18

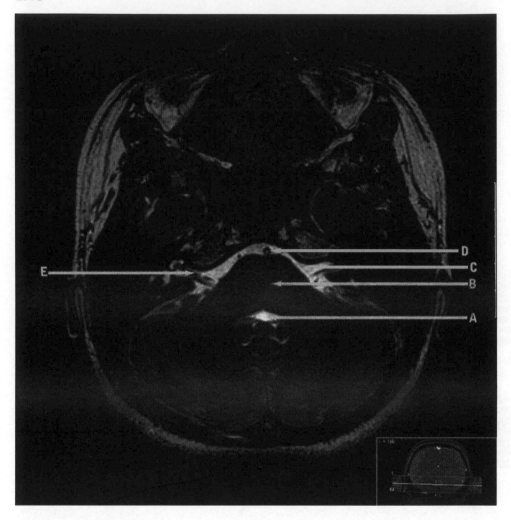

Answer the following questions.

1   Name structure 'A'.
2   Which cranial nerves arise from 'B'?
3   Name structure 'C'.
4   Name structure 'D'.
5   Name structure 'E'.

2.19

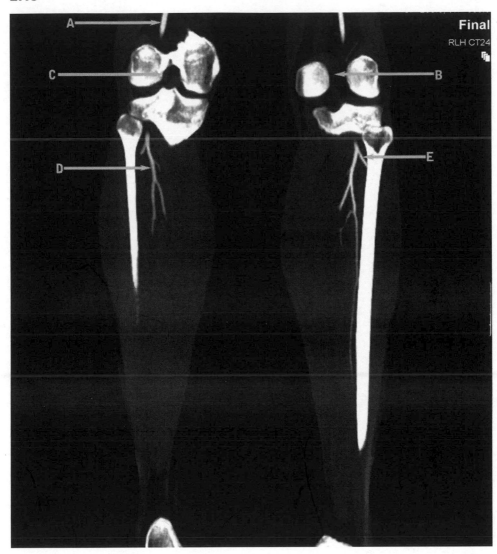

Answer the following questions.

1 Name structure 'A'.
2 Name structure 'B'.
3 Which structure attaches to 'C'?
4 Name structure 'D'.
5 Name structure 'E'.

2.20

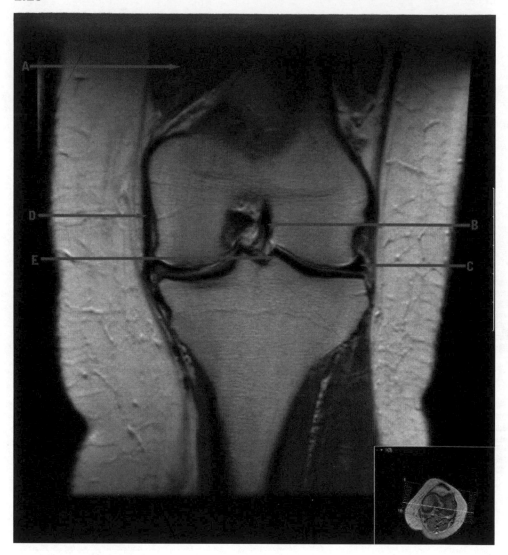

Answer the following questions.

1   Name structure 'A'.
2   Name structure 'B'.
3   Name structure 'C'.
4   Name structure 'D'.
5   Name structure 'E'.

Answers

2.1

1 Lateral Malleolus of Fibula.
2 Peroneus Longus Muscle.
3 Peroneus Brevis Tendon.
4 Cuboid Bone.
5 Abductor Digiti Minimi Muscle.

Parasagittal MRI ankle.

The presence of the smaller fibula indicates this is the lateral ankle. The peroneus brevis and longus tendons run behind the lateral malleolus. Peroneus brevis is shorter, can be seen running in front of peroneus longus and inserts in the base of the 5th metatarsal.

2.2

1 Left Body of Mandible.
2 Epiglottis.
3 Left Vallecula.
4 Right Thyroid Cartilage.
5 Left Pyriform Fossa.

Double contrast barium swallow – larynx.

The valleculae and pyriform fossae can be seen. The pyriform fossae are important structures in the diagnosis of neck malignancy and therefore knowledge of this normal anatomical appearance is important. Subtle irregularities in the shape of these potential spaces may indicate neoplasm.

2.3

1 Diaphysis of Left Femur.
2 Left Patella.
3 Left Fabella.
4 Left Suprapatellar Fat Pad.
5 Left Patellar Tendon.

Lateral knee radiograph.

Note the side marker. The fabella is a sesamoid bone found in the tendon of the lateral head of gastrocnemius behind the lateral femoral condyle.

The patellar tendon is the continuation of the central portion of the quadriceps tendon – it inserts at the tibial tuberosity.

2.4
1   T12.
2   Gastroduodenal Artery.
3   Common Hepatic Artery.
4   Superior Mesenteric Artery.
5   Left Iliacus Muscle.

Coronal CT angiogram of mesenteric vessels.

The coeliac artery is identified by its 'seagull' appearance at the bifurcation, forming the splenic and common hepatic arteries. Prior to this, and often difficult to identify, is the origin of the left gastric artery. The superior mesenteric artery (SMA) can be seen supplying the jejunum and ileum.

2.5
1   Clivus.
2   Pons.
3   Splenium of Corpus Callosum.
4   Cingulate Gyrus.
5   Optic Chiasma in Suprasellar Cistern.

Sagittal T1W MRI brain.

The high signal within the clivus is due to the presence of bone marrow. Loss of this high signal may indicate pathology. Further high signal is seen within the pituitary fossa – a normal finding thought to be due to the presence of antidiuretic hormone (ADH) **neurosecretory granule**s.

2.6
1   Jejunum.
2   Terminal Ileum.
3   Transverse Colon.
4   Caecum.
5   Right Sacroiliac Joint.

Single contrast barium follow-through study.

The jejunum has a 'fluffy' appearance and is slightly wider in calibre, differentiating it from ileum.

2.7
1   Left Sternocleidomastoid Muscle.
2   Left Common Carotid Artery.
3   Isthmus of Thyroid Gland.
4   Trachea.
5   Left Lobe of Thyroid Gland.

Transverse US thyroid gland – high frequency transducer.

Convention dictates that this is the left lobe. The internal jugular vein, being a venous structure, is compressible and can be seen lateral to the common carotid artery. The trachea is seen due to the 'ring down' artefact produced by gas within it.

2.8

1   Right Femoral Artery.
2   Left Obturator Internus Muscle.
3   Left Ischio-anal Fossa.
4   Right Obturator Externus Muscle.
5   Left Gluteus Maximus Muscle.

Axial T1W MRI female pelvis.

The urethra and vagina are visible. The signal void produced by fast flowing blood in the femoral artery indicates this is an arterial rather than venous structure.

The ischioanal fossa is an important structure in pelvic sepsis and involvement can be readily identified on contrast enhanced MRI.

2.9

1   Left side of Quadrigeminal Plate.
2   Left Head of Caudate Nucleus.
3   Septum Pellucidum.
4   3rd Ventricle.
5   Anterior Limb of Right Internal Capsule.

Axial CT brain.

Grey matter structures such as the cerebral cortex and basal ganglia are seen as relatively higher attenuation structures whereas white matter tracts such as the internal capsule are of a lower attenuation – this is partly due to the differences in physical density between them.

Identification of the cerebrospinal fluid (CSF) spaces and any asymmetry is essential in interpreting CT studies of the brain.

2.10

1   Right Lower Lobe Bronchus.
2   Right Internal Thoracic Artery.
3   Left Pulmonary Vein.
4   Left Basal Pulmonary Artery.
5   Thecal Sac.

Axial contrast enhanced CT chest.

When read in an anteroposterior direction, the hilar structures are:

> Right hemithorax: Pulmonary **V**ein, Pulmonary **A**rtery, **B**ronchus – **VAB**
> Left hemithorax: Pulmonary **V**ein, **B**ronchus, Pulmonary **A**rtery – **VBA.**

The internal thoracic artery (ITA) is also known as the internal mammary artery (IMA) and is used in Coronary Artery Bypass surgery.

2.11
1 Base of 1st **Metacarpal**.
2 **Capitate Bone**.
3 Scaphoid Bone.
4 Triangular Fibrocartilage Complex.
5 Ulnar Styloid.

Dorsopalmar MRI hand.

2.12
1 Right Coracoid Process.
2 Posterior Aspect of Right 1st Rib.
3 Medial Border of Right Scapula.
4 Greater Tuberosity of Right Humerus.
5 Inferior Aspect of Right Glenoid.

Frontal shoulder radiograph.

The scapula and ribs should be inspected for injury in cases of shoulder girdle pain or trauma. The acromioclavicular, coracoclavicular and acromiohumeral distances can be clearly seen.

Alteration of these measurements should raise suspicion of pathology.

2.13
1 Right Incudomalleolar Complex.
2 Left Hypoglossal Nerve.
3 Os Terminale.
4 Left Lateral Mass of C2 Vertebral Body.
5 Trachea.

Coronal CT neck – bone windows.

The os terminale – a secondary ossification centre – usually fuses to form the normal dens in childhood. It rarely remains unfused, as in this case, and may be misinterpreted as a fracture. It can be seen however that C2 and the os are well corticated, aiding differentiation from traumatic injury.

This coronal image is the CT equivalent of the 'peg view' radiograph obtained in cervical trauma. The C1/C2 lateral mass alignment and dens integrity can be inspected.

2.14
1 Superior Mesenteric Vein and Splenic Vein.
2 Inferior Vena Cava.
3 Right Crus of Diaphragm.
4 Stomach.
5 Left Adrenal Gland.

Axial MRI abdomen.

Absence of signal is seen in vascular structures as well as the stomach due to its gas content. The diaphragmatic crura and retrocrural space (containing high signal fat) can be identified.

2.15
1 Portal Vein.
2 Splenic Vein.
3 Superior Mesenteric Artery.
4 Abdominal Aorta.
5 Vertebral Body.

Transverse US abdomen – low frequency transducer.

Identification of these structures by obtaining this image is routine in abdominal sonography.

The portal vessels have a hyperechoic wall on US, differentiating them from the hepatic veins.

The vertebral body is identified due to the posterior acoustic shadowing it produces.

2.16
1 Vomer.
2 Left Lateral Pterygoid Plate.
3 Left Mandibular Condyle.
4 Right Mastoid Air Cells.
5 Internal Occipital Protuberance.

Axial CT base of skull – bone windows.

The absence of signal from the gas containing sinuses can be helpful – the presence of fluid density opacity in the mastoid air cells or maxillary antra can indicate base of skull or facial fractures respectively.

2.17
1 Median Glossoepiglottic Fold.
2 Left Submandibular Gland.
3 Right Common Carotid Artery.
4 Right Vertebral Artery.
5 Right Inferior Oblique Muscle.

Axial contrast enhanced CT neck.

2.18
1 4th Ventricle.
2 Cranial Nerves V – VIII.
3 Left Internal Auditory Meatus.
4 Basilar Artery.
5 Right Facial Nerve (Cranial Nerve VII).

Axial T2W MRI of internal auditory meatus (IAM).

CN VII and the cochlear portion of CN VIII lie anterior to the superior and inferior vestibular portions of CN VIII.

This sequence allows identification of any cerebellopontine angle masses – the commonest of which is the vestibular schwannoma.

2.19
1   Right Popliteal Artery.
2   Medial Head of Left Gastrocnemius.
3   Right Anterior Cruciate Ligament.
4   Right Tibioperoneal Trunk.
5   Left Anterior Tibial Artery.

Coronal CT angiogram lower limb vessels.

The popliteal artery trifurcates into the anterior and posterior tibial and peroneal arteries. In many cases a short tibioperoneal trunk is seen after the origin of the anterior tibial artery.

The anterior tibial is identified due to its proximal origin and relatively lateral course.

2.20
1   Vastus Medialis Muscle.
2   Anterior Cruciate Ligament.
3   Lateral Meniscus.
4   Medial Collateral Ligament.
5   Lateral Intercondylar Tubercle.

Coronal T1W MRI knee.

There are no side markers however convention would dictate that this is the left knee due to the presence of the fibula and the site of the popliteus tendon insertion on the lateral femoral condyle. The anterior cruciate ligament (ACL) has a relatively more horizontal course than the posterior cruciate ligament (PCL) and can be seen inserting into the medial border of the lateral femoral condyle.

Exam 3

3.1

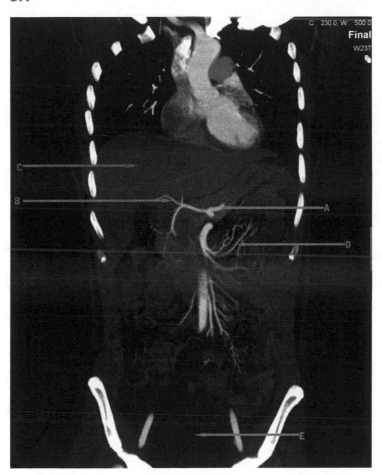

Answer the following questions.

1   Name structure 'A'.
2   Name structure 'B'.
3   Name structure 'C'.
4   Name structure 'D'.
5   Name structure 'E'.

3.2

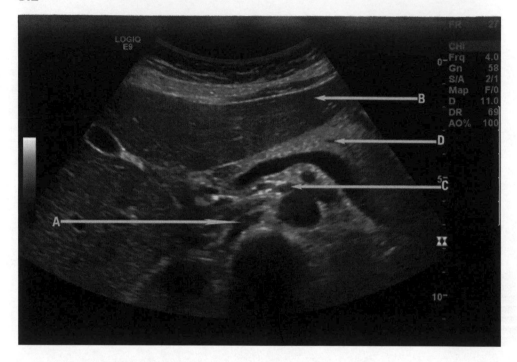

Answer the following questions.

1   Name structure 'A'.
2   Name structure 'B'.
3   Name structure 'C'.
4   Name structure 'D'.
5   What is the calibre of 'D' in the head of the pancreas?

3.3

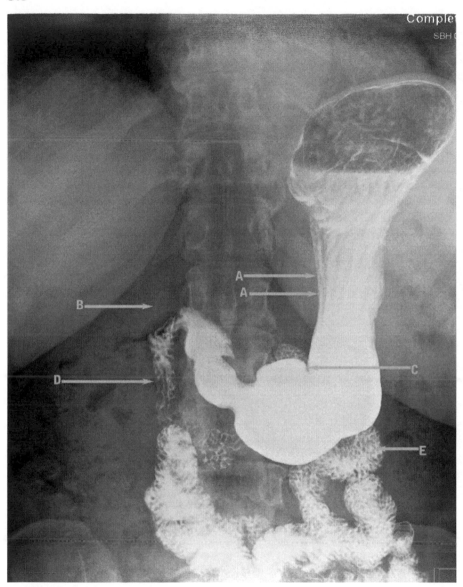

Answer the following questions.

1 Name structure 'A'.
2 Name structure 'B'.
3 Name structure 'C'.
4 Name structure 'D'.
5 Name structure 'E'.

3.4

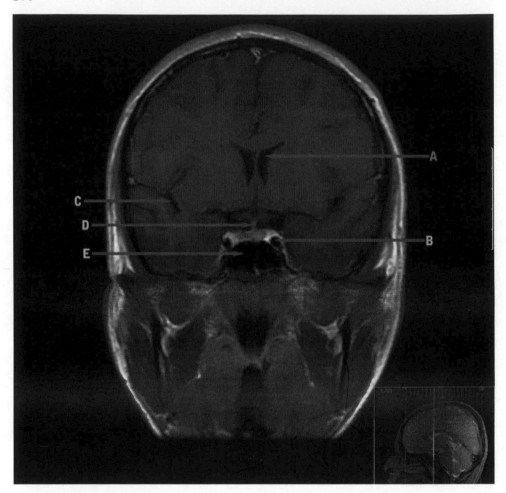

Answer the following questions.

1   Name structure 'A'.
2   Name structure 'B'.
3   Name structure 'C'.
4   Name structure 'D'.
5   Name structure 'E'.

3.5

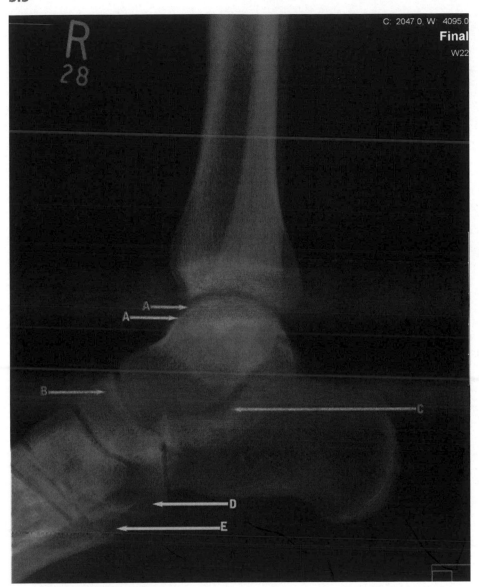

Answer the following questions.

1 Name structure 'A'.
2 Name structure 'B'.
3 Name structure 'C'.
4 Name structure 'D'.
5 Name structure 'E'.

3.6

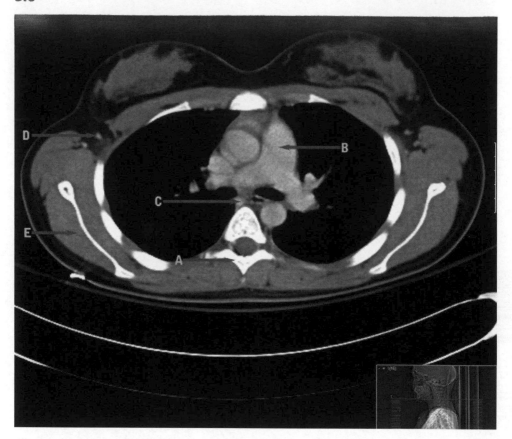

Answer the following questions.

1   Name structure 'A'.
2   Name structure 'B'.
3   Name structure 'C'.
4   Name structure 'D'.
5   Name structure 'E'.

3.7

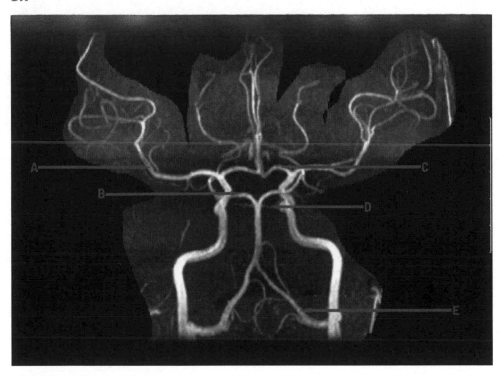

Answer the following questions.

1   Name structure 'A'.
2   Name structure 'B'.
3   Name structure 'C'.
4   Name structure 'D'.
5   Name structure 'E'.

3.8

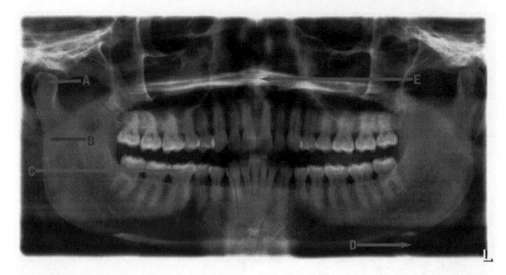

Answer the following questions.

1   Name structure 'A'.
2   Name structure 'B'.
3   Name structure 'C'.
4   Name structure 'D'.
5   Name structure 'E'.

3.9

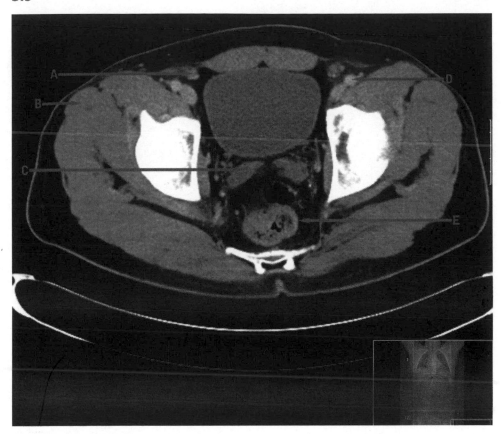

Answer the following questions.

1   Name structure 'A'.
2   Name structure 'B'.
3   Name structure 'C'.
4   Name structure 'D'.
5   Which fascial structure separates 'C' from 'E'?

3.10

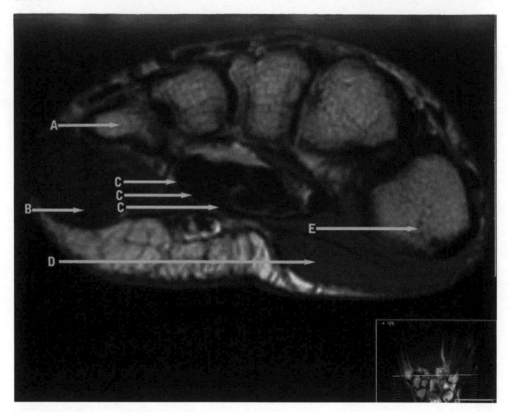

Answer the following questions.

1　Name structure 'A'.
2　Name structure 'B'.
3　Name structure 'C'.
4　Name structure 'D'.
5　Name structure 'E'.

3.11

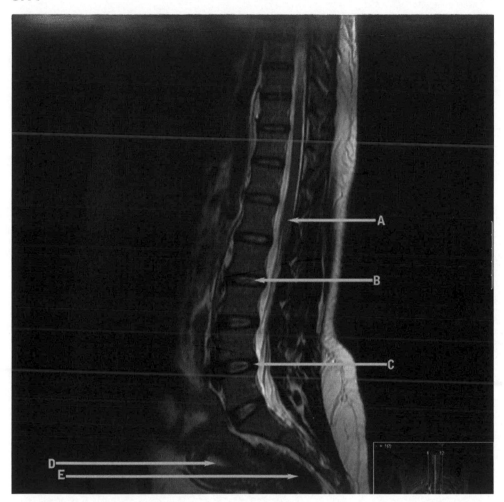

Answer the following questions.

1   Name structure 'A'.
2   Name structure 'B'.
3   Name structure 'C'.
4   Name structure 'D'.
5   Name structure 'E'.

3.12

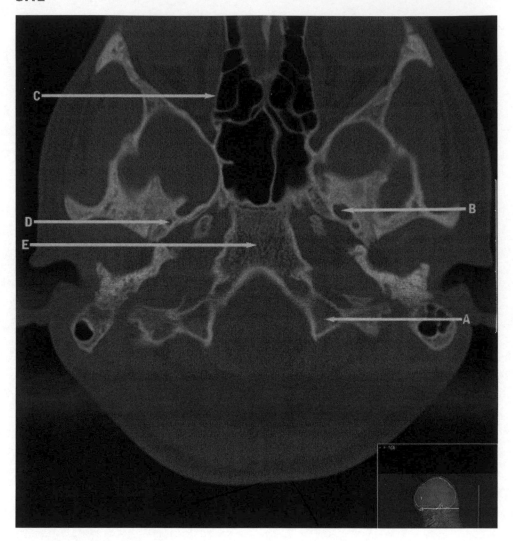

Answer the following questions.

1   Name structure 'A'.
2   Name structure 'B'.
3   Name structure 'C'.
4   Which vascular structures pass through 'D'?
5   Name structure 'E'.

3.13

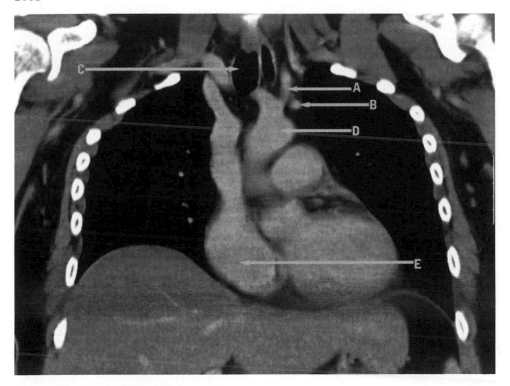

Answer the following questions.

1   Name structure 'A'.
2   Name structure 'B'.
3   Name structure 'C'.
4   Name structure 'D'.
5   Name structure 'E'.

3.14

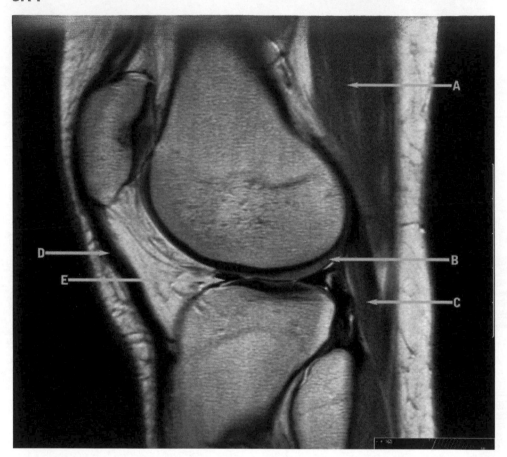

Answer the following questions.

1   Name structure 'A'.
2   Name structure 'B'.
3   Name structure 'C'.
4   Name structure 'D'.
5   Name structure 'E'.

3.15

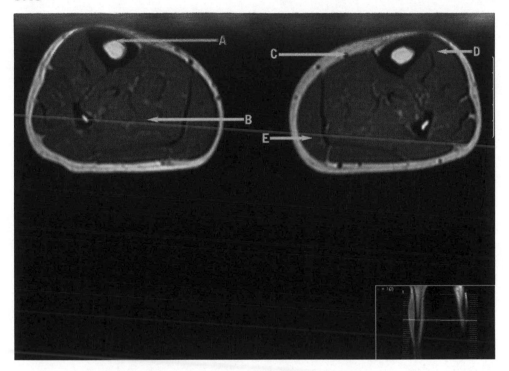

Answer the following questions.

1   Name structure 'A'.
2   Name structure 'B'.
3   Name structure 'C'.
4   Name structure 'D'.
5   Name structure 'E'.

3.16

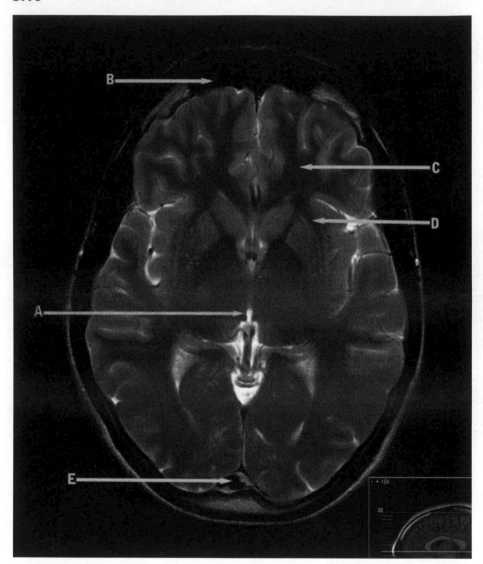

Answer the following questions.

1   Name structure 'A'.
2   Name structure 'B'.
3   Name structure 'C'.
4   Name structure 'D'.
5   Name structure 'E'.

3.17

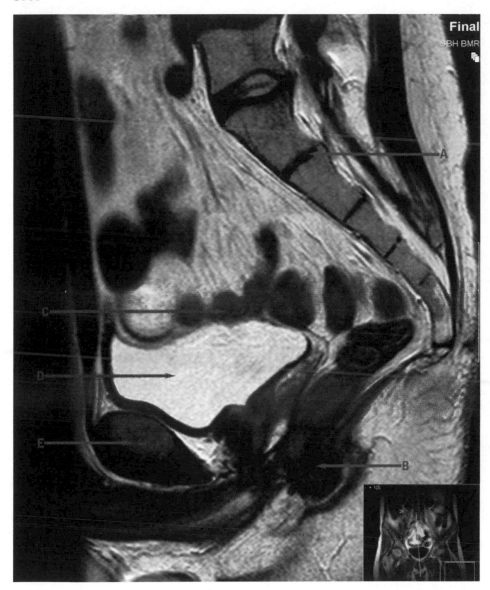

Answer the following questions.

1 Name structure 'A'.
2 Name structure 'B'.
3 Name structure 'C'.
4 Name structure 'D'.
5 Name structure 'E'.

3.18

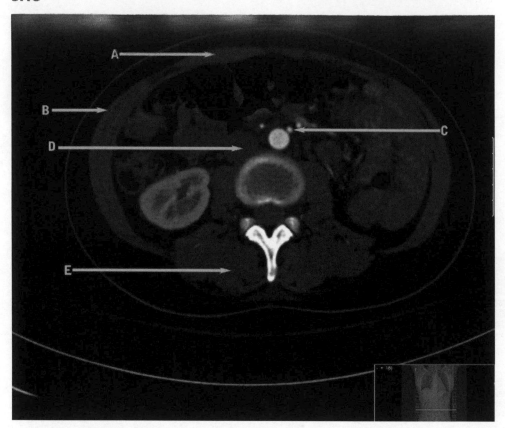

Answer the following questions.

1 Name structure 'A'.
2 Name structure 'B'.
3 Name structure 'C'.
4 Name structure 'D'.
5 Name structure 'E'.

3.19

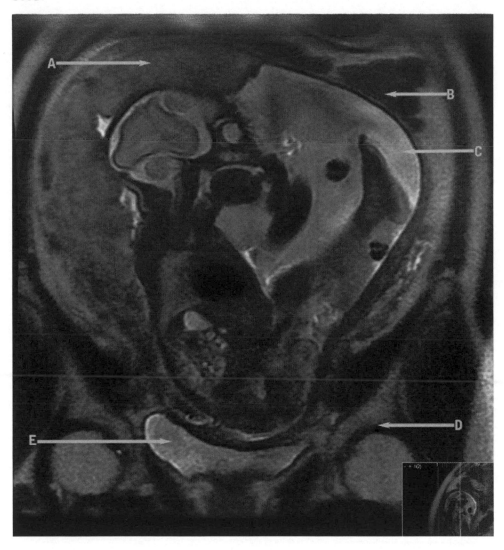

MRI Foetus – Answer the following questions.

1   Name structure 'A'.
2   Name structure 'B'.
3   Name structure 'C'.
4   Name structure 'D'.
5   Name structure 'E'.

3.20

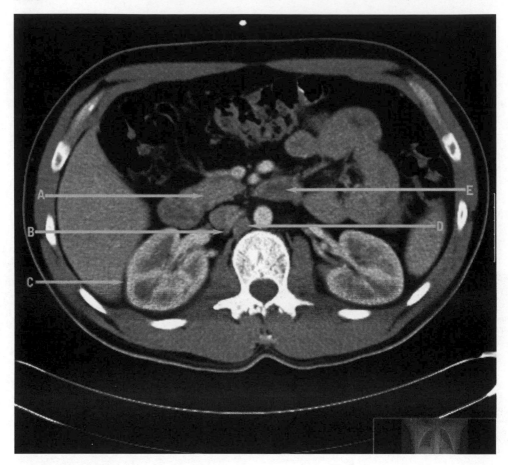

Answer the following questions.

1   Name structure 'A'.
2   Name structure 'B'.
3   What is the name of the peritoneal space at 'C'?
4   Name structure 'D'.
5   Name structure 'E'.

Answers

3.1
1. Splenic Artery.
2. True Hepatic Artery.
3. Right Lobe of Liver.
4. Jejunal Branches of SMA.
5. Urinary Bladder.

Coronal CT angiogram mesenteric vessels.

The bifurcation of the common hepatic artery, forming the hepatic and gastroduodenal (GDA) arteries is seen. The true hepatic further divides into left and right hepatic arteries. The GDA is frequently involved in cases of non variceal upper gastrointestinal haemorrhage – an understanding of its normal course and appearance is therefore important.

3.2
1. Inferior Vena Cava.
2. Left Lobe of Liver.
3. Left Renal Vein.
4. Pancreatic Duct.
5. 3mm.

Transverse US abdomen – low frequency transducer.

The pancreatic duct is seen within the body of the pancreas. The pancreas may appear hyperechoic ('bright') on US, or in thin or elderly patients, relatively hypoechoic. The bright appearance is due to the presence of highly reflective fat. On transverse abdominal US, the pancreas is seen lying anterior to the splenic vein.

3.3
1. Lesser Curvature of Stomach.
2. Right Transverse Process of L1.
3. Incisura.
4. D2.
5. Jejunum.

Single contrast barium study.

This erect image is taken at the end of a routine barium swallow study and is used to identify gross pathology of the gastric fundus which may cause symptoms. The normal course of the duodenum can be seen:

> **D1:** The duodenal cap or bulb – a continuation of the pylorus which passes posterolaterally and superiorly

D2: Passes inferiorly

D3: The horizontal segment which crosses the midline

D4: Ascends to the left L2 pedicle/transverse process, to the duodenojejunal flexure, at the ligament of Treitz.

D1–D3 form a 'C' loop within which lies the head of the pancreas. The latter part of D1, D2, D3 and D4 are retroperitoneal.

3.4

1 Left Lateral Ventricle.
2 Cavernous Internal Carotid Artery.
3 Right Sylvian Fissure or Lateral Sulcus.
4 Pituitary Infundibulum.
5 Sphenoid Sinus.

Coronal T1W MRI brain.

Various classifications exist for the segments of the ICA. One commonly used system is:

> **Cervical ICA –** within the neck
> **Petrous ICA –** including its passage through the foramen lacerum
> **Cavernous ICA –** within the cavernous sinus
> **Supraclinoid ICA –** it then pierces the dura mater and terminates at the Circle of Willis.

3.5

1 Dome of Right Talus.
2 Right Navicular Bone.
3 Sinus Tarsi of Right Ankle.
4 Right Cuboid Bone.
5 Base of Right 5th Metatarsal.

Lateral ankle radiograph.

3.6

1 Right Lamina of Vertebral Body.
2 Pulmonary Trunk.
3 Azygos Vein.
4 Right Axillary Vessels.
5 Right Infraspinatus Muscle.

Axial contrast enhanced CT chest.

The axillary artery and vein cannot be reliably distinguished here. The azygos vein is formed by the ascending lumbar veins and rises in the posterior mediastinum until it arches over the right main bronchus to drain into the SVC.

3.7

1   **Right Middle Cerebral Artery.**
2   **Right Posterior Cerebral Artery.**
3   Left Anterior Cerebral Artery.
4   Left Superior Cerebellar Artery.
5   Left Vertebral Artery.

Reformatted MR angiogram circle of Willis (CoW).

The genu of the middle cerebral artery (MCA) indicates the junction of M1 and M2 segments. M1 supplies the basal ganglia via the lenticulostriate perforating end arteries. Occlusion causes lacunar strokes, commonly identified on CT.

3.8

1   Right Mandibular Condyle.
2   Right Mandibular Ramus.
3   Right Lower 1st Molar.
4   Hyoid Bone (Left).
5   Hard Palate.

Orthopantomogram (OPG).

Full complement of incisors, canines, premolars and molars is seen.

3.9

1   Right Spermatic Cord.
2   Right Tensor Fasciae Latae Muscle.
3   Right Seminal Vesicle.
4   Left Femoral Artery.
5   Denonvillier's Fascia.

Axial contrast enhanced CT male pelvis.

Denonvillier's fascia, also known as the rectovesical fascia, separates the anterior bladder, prostate and seminal vesicles from the posterior rectum. This is removed, along with the mesorectal fascia in total mesorectal excision, in cases of rectal malignancy.

3.10

1   Hamate Bone.
2   Abductor Digiti Minimi Muscle.
3   Flexor Retinaculum.
4   Abductor Pollicis Brevis Muscle.
5   Base of 1st Metacarpal.

Axial MRI hand.

The flexor retinaculum is seen to surround the flexor tendons of the hand.

The ulnar vessels and nerve are seen volar to the flexor retinaculum.

The hamate is identified due to the presence of its 'hook'.

3.11
1 Conus Medullaris.
2 Nucleus Pulposus of L2/3 Intervertebral Disc.
3 Annulus Fibrosus of L4/5 Intervertebral Disc.
4 Endometrium of Uterus.
5 Rectum.

Sagittal MRI lumbosacral spine.

The zonal anatomy of the uterus can be seen:

> **Endometrium** – high signal
> **Inner myometrium (junctional zone)** – low signal
> **Outer myometrium** – intermediate signal.

The normal intranuclear cleft can be seen in the L2/3 – L5/S1 discs. The appearance of this cleft may be lost when an inflammatory process affects the intervertebral disc.

3.12
1 Left Occipital Condyle.
2 Left Foramen Ovale.
3 **Right Lamina Papyracea.**
4 Right Middle Meningeal Artery and Vein.
5 Clivus.

Axial CT base of skull – bone windows.

Several skull base foramina can be identified. The foramen lacerum, through which passes the petrous portion of the ICA, lies posteromedial to the foramen ovale and foramen spinosum.

3.13
1 Left Common Carotid Artery.
2 Left Subclavian Artery.
3 Trachea.
4 Aortic Arch.
5 Right Atrium.

Coronal contrast enhanced CT chest.

The right atrium forms the right heart border. The left ventricle and left ventricular outflow tract are seen.

3.14
1 Biceps Femoris Muscle.
2 Articular Cartilage of Femur.
3 Lateral Head of Gastrocnemius.
4 Patellar Tendon.
5 Anterior Horn of Lateral Menicus.

Sagittal T1W MRI knee.

3.15

1   Right Tibia.
2   Right Soleus Muscle.
3   Left Long Saphenous Vein.
4   Left Tibialis Anterior Muscle.
5   Medial Head of Left Gastrocnemius.

Axial MRI lower limbs.

The aponeurosis of the gastrocnemius muscles can be seen as a band separating the medial and lateral heads.

3.16

1   3rd Ventricle.
2   Right Frontal Sinus.
3   White Matter of Left Frontal Lobe.
4   Left External Capsule.
5   Confluence of Venous Sinuses (Torcular Herophili).

Axial T2W MRI brain.

Posterior to the caudate nucleus lies the lentiform nucleus, composed of the medial globus pallidus and lateral putamen.

High signal CSF is seen in the 3rd ventricle and trigone of the lateral ventricles.

The confluence of venous sinuses, formed by the superior sagittal sinus and straight sinus, is seen as it diverges, forming the transverse sinuses.

3.17

1   Intervertebral Disc of S1/2.
2   Rectum.
3   Ileum.
4   Urinary Bladder.
5   Pubic Symphysis.

Sagittal T2W MRI male pelvis.

3.18

1   Right Rectus Abdominis Muscle.
2   Right External Oblique Muscle.
3   Inferior Mesenteric Artery.
4   Inferior Vena Cava.
5   Right Erector Spinae Muscle.

Axial contrast enhanced CT abdomen.

Branches of the SMA are also visible, as are the facet joints between vertebral bodies.

3.19

1   **Placenta.**
2   **Small Bowel.**
3   Amniotic Fluid.
4   Left Acetabulum.
5   Urinary Bladder.

Coronal MRI foetus.

The foetal heart is seen as low signal anterior to the higher signal, fluid containing foetal lung. Cerebral structures and the umbilical cord within the amniotic sac can also be identified.

3.20

1   Head of Pancreas.
2   Right Renal Artery.
3   Hepatorenal Recess – Morison's Pouch.
4   Right Crus of Diaphragm.
5   D3 – Horizontal Segment of Duodenum.

Axial contrast enhanced CT abdomen.

The common bile duct is seen within the head of the pancreas, and lateral to this is the 2nd part of the duodenum. The normal anatomical relationship of the superior mesenteric vein (SMV) and SMA, reversed in malrotation, is seen. The SMV lies to the right and lateral to the SMA.

Exam 4

4.1

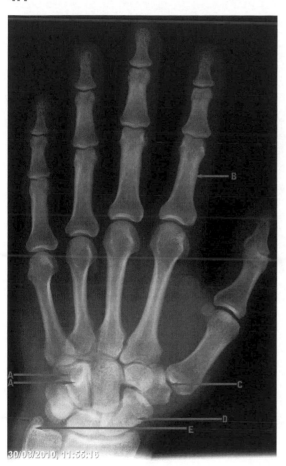

Answer the following questions.

1   Name structure 'A'.
2   Name structure 'B'.
3   Name structure 'C'.
4   Name structure 'D'.
5   Which ligament attaches to 'E'?

4.2

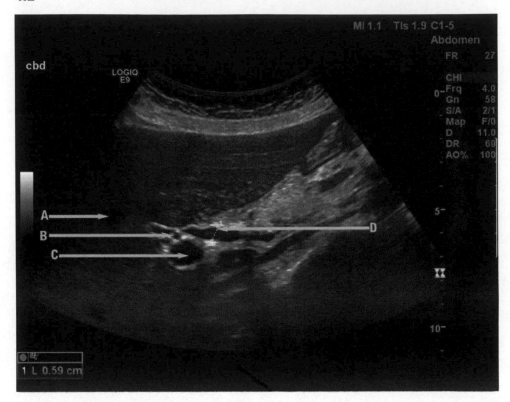

Answer the following questions.

1   Name structure 'A'.
2   Name structure 'B'.
3   Name structure 'C'.
4   Name structure 'D'.
5   Where does structure 'D' terminate?

4.3

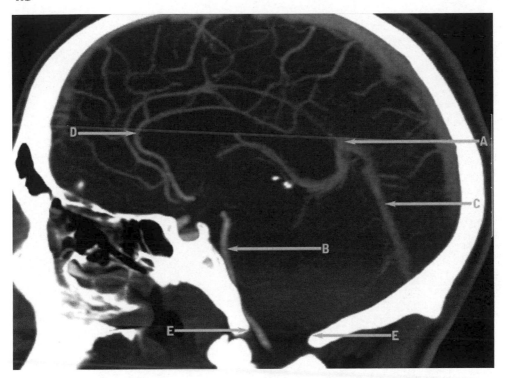

Answer the following questions.

1 Name structure 'A'.
2 Name structure 'B'.
3 Name structure 'C'.
4 Name structure 'D'.
5 What is the name given to space bounded by 'E'?

4.4

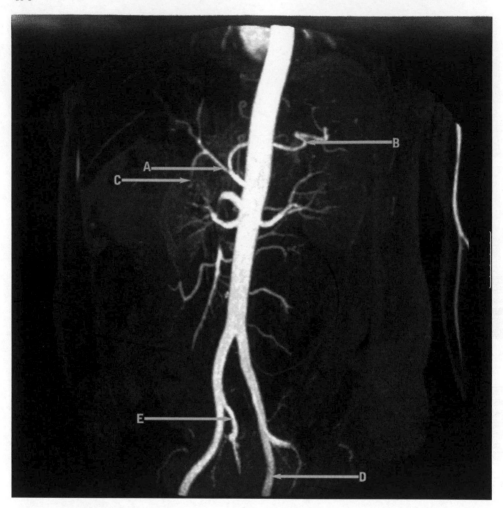

Answer the following questions.

1 Name structure 'A'.
2 Name structure 'B'.
3 What are the branches of 'C'?
4 Name structure 'D'.
5 Name structure 'E'.

4.5

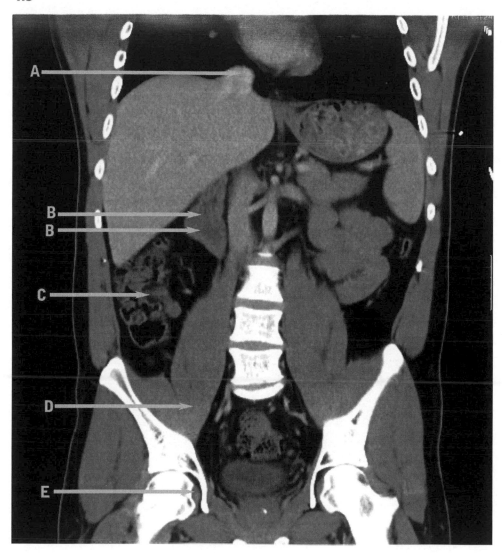

Answer the following questions.

1 At what level does 'A' pierce the diaphragm?
2 Name structure 'B'.
3 Name structure 'C'.
4 Name structure 'D'.
5 Which structure attaches at 'E'?

4.6

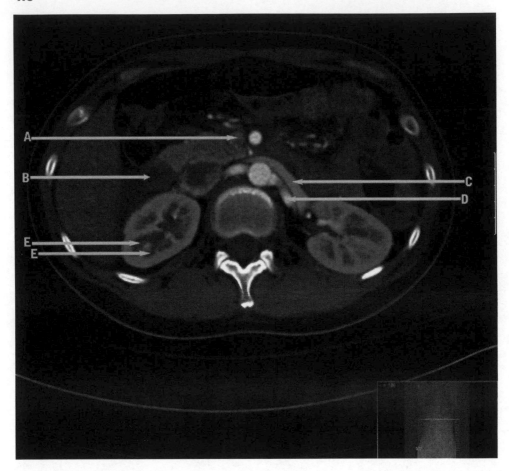

Answer the following questions.

1   Name structure 'A'.
2   Name structure 'B'.
3   Name structure 'C'.
4   Name structure 'D'.
5   Name structure 'E'.

4.7

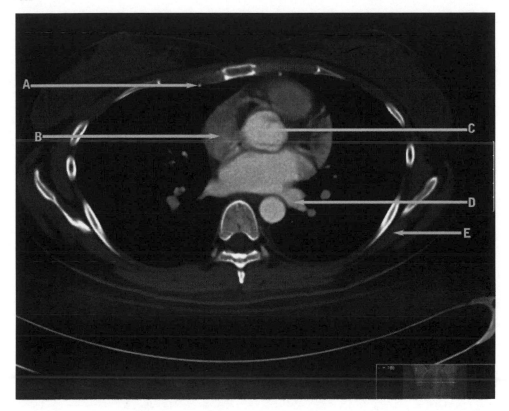

Answer the following questions.

1 What is the origin of 'A'?
2 Name structure 'B'.
3 Name structure 'C'.
4 Name structure 'D'.
5 Name structure 'E'.

4.8

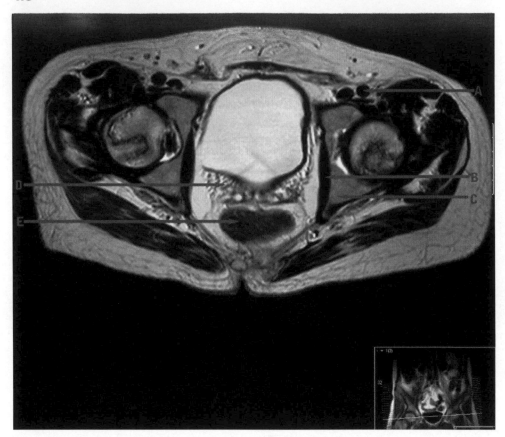

Answer the following questions.

1   Name structure 'A'.
2   Name structure 'B'.
3   Name structure 'C'.
4   Where does structure 'D' drain?
5   Name structure 'E'.

4.9

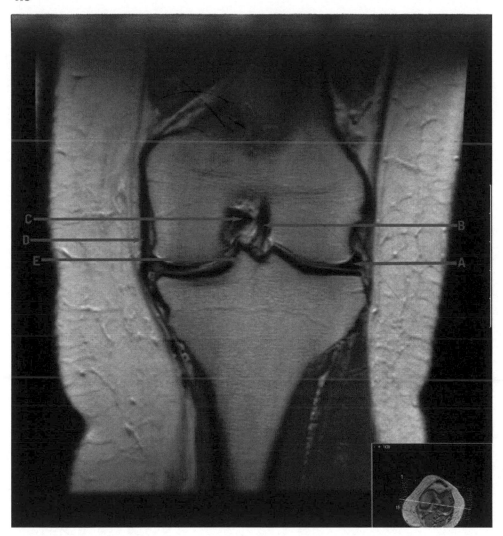

Answer the following questions.

1 Which tendon is found adjacent to 'A'?
2 Name structure 'B'.
3 Name structure 'C'.
4 Name structure 'D'.
5 Name structure 'E'.

4.10

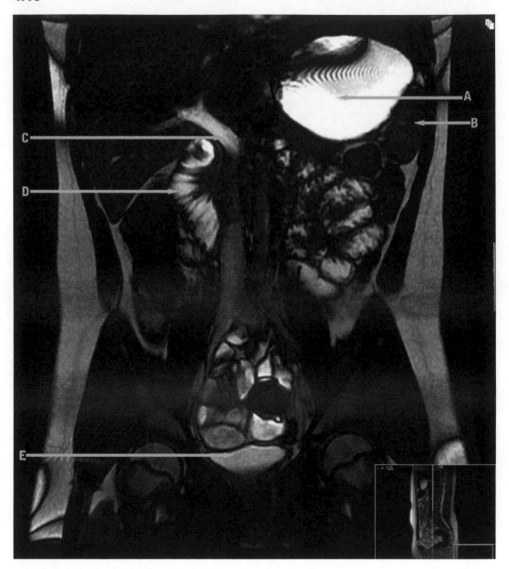

Answer the following questions.

1   Name structure 'A'.
2   Name structure 'B'.
3   Name structure 'C'.
4   Name structure 'D'.
5   Name structure 'E'.

4.11

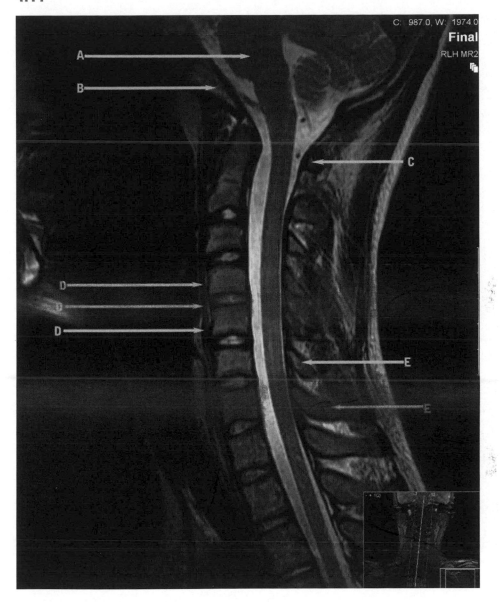

Answer the following questions.

1   Name structure 'A'.
2   Name structure 'B'.
3   Name structure 'C'.
4   Name structure 'D'.
5   Which structure lies between 'E' and 'E'?

4.12

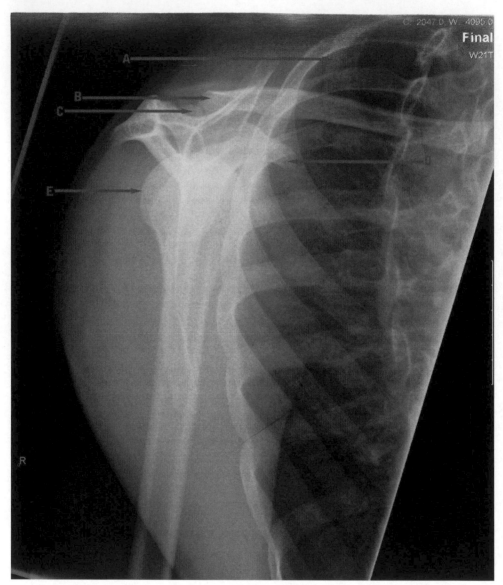

Answer the following questions.

1   With which structure does 'A' articulate?
2   Name structure 'B'.
3   Name structure 'C'.
4   Name structure 'D'.
5   Which component of the rotator cuff is found at 'E'?

4.13

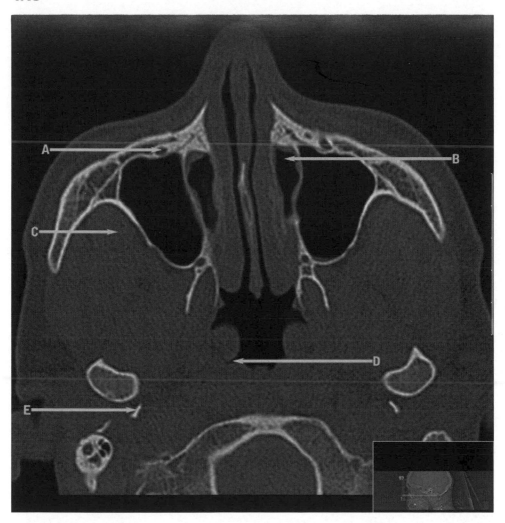

Answer the following questions.

1 Name structure 'A'.
2 Name structure 'B'.
3 Name structure 'C'.
4 Name structure 'D'.
5 Name structure 'E'.

4.14

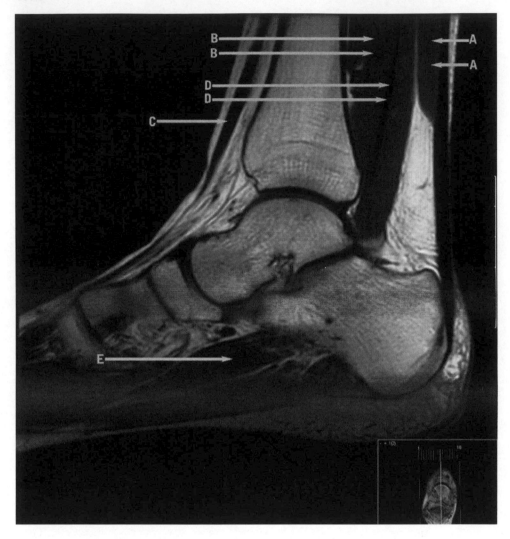

Answer the following questions.

1 Name structure 'A'.
2 Name structure 'B'.
3 Name structure 'C'.
4 Name structure 'D'.
5 Name structure 'E'.

4.15

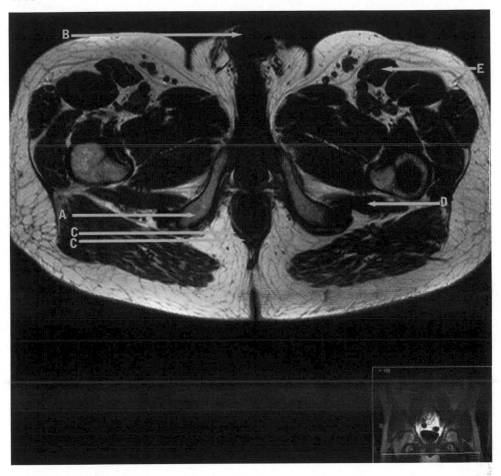

Answer the following questions.

1 Name structure 'A'.
2 Name structure 'B'.
3 Name structure 'C'.
4 Name structure 'D'.
5 Name structure 'E'.

4.16

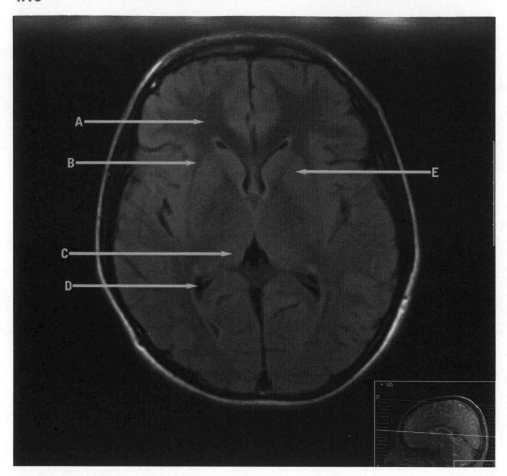

Answer the following questions.

1 Name structure 'A'.
2 Name structure 'B'.
3 Name structure 'C'.
4 Name structure 'D'.
5 Which end arteries supply 'E'?

4.17

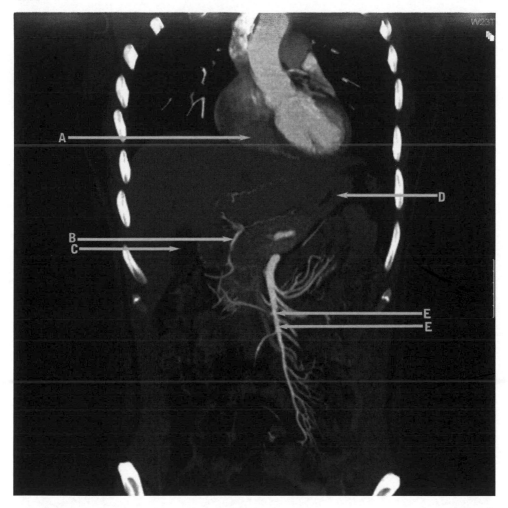

Answer the following questions.

1 Name structure 'A'.
2 Name structure 'B'.
3 Name structure 'C'.
4 Name structure 'D'.
5 At which vertebral level does 'E' arise?

4.18

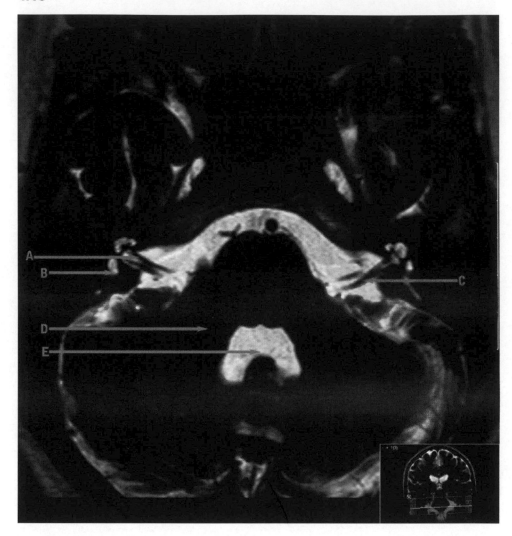

Answer the following questions.

1   Name structure 'A'.
2   Name structure 'B'.
3   Name structure 'C'.
4   Name structure 'D'.
5   Name structure 'E'.

4.19

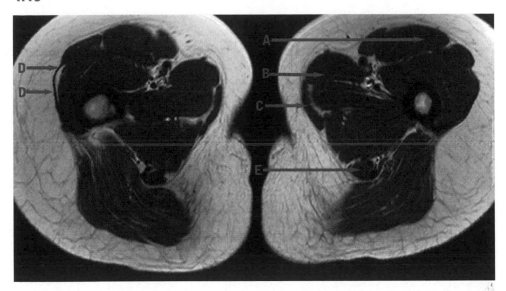

Answer the following questions.

1   Name structure 'A'.
2   Name structure 'B'.
3   Name structure 'C'.
4   Name structure 'D'.
5   **Name structure 'E'.**

4.20

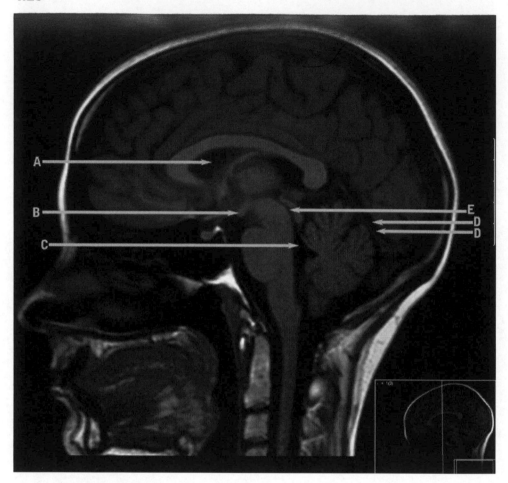

Answer the following questions.

1 Name structure 'A'.
2 Name structure 'B'.
3 Name structure 'C'.
4 Name structure 'D'.
5 Name structure 'E'.

Answers

4.1
1   Hook of Hamate Bone.
2   Diaphysis of Proximal Phalanx of Index Finger.
3   1st Carpometacarpal Joint.
4   Scaphoid Bone.
5   Ulnar Collateral Ligament.

Dorsopalmar wrist radiograph.

4.2
1   Hepatic Vein.
2   Hepatic Artery.
3   Portal Vein.
4   Common Bile Duct.
5   Hepatopancreatic Ampulla at D2 (Ampulla of Vater).

Subcostal US abdomen.

Although the appearance of the abdominal organs is variable, this image demonstrates an almost universal finding – the portal vein and the anterior common bile duct (CBD), with the hepatic artery in transverse between. The size of the CBD varies with age and increases post cholecystectomy. Accurate measurement is essential as changes in calibre can indicate a range of pathology. Colour Doppler reveals an absence of flow in this structure, arterial flow in the hepatic artery, and constant or phasic flow in the portal vein.

4.3
1   Great Cerebral Vein of Galen.
2   Basilar Artery.
3   Straight Sinus.
4   Anterior Cerebral Artery.
5   Foramen Magnum.

Sagittal CT cerebral angiogram.

The venous contamination in this study demonstrates the internal cerebral veins joining with the basal vein of Rosenthal to form the vein of Galen.

4.4
1   Common Hepatic Artery.
2   Splenic Artery.
3   Superior Pancreaticoduodenal Artery and Right Gastroepiploic Artery.
4   Left External Iliac Artery.
5   Right Internal Iliac Artery.

Reformat of MR angiogram abdominal aorta.

4.5

1   T8.
2   D2 – 2nd Part of Duodenum.
3   Ileocaecal Valve.
4   Right Iliopsoas Muscle.
5   Right Ligamentum Teres Femoris.

Coronal contrast enhanced CT abdomen.

The iliopsoas muscle is formed by psoas major, minor and the iliacus muscles. It inserts at the lesser trochanter of the femur. The fovea capitis is the rounded depression within the head of femur where the ligamentum teres attaches.

4.6

1   Superior Mesenteric Vein.
2   D2 – 2nd Part of Duodenum.
3   Left Renal Vein.
4   Left Renal Artery.
5   Medulla of Right Kidney.

Axial CT angiogram of abdomen.

The relationship of SMV to SMA is demonstrated. This arterial phase study demonstrates the enhancement of the renal cortex.

4.7

1   Right Subclavian Artery.
2   **Right Atrium**.
3   **Aortic Root/Valve**.
4   Left Inferior Pulmonary Vein.
5   Left Trapezius Muscle.

Axial contrast enhanced CT chest.

4.8

1   Left External Iliac Artery.
2   Left Obturator Internus Muscle.
3   Left Ischium.
4   Right Vas Deferens.
5   Rectum.

Axial T2W MRI male pelvis.

The seminal vesicles are seen as high signal due to their fluid content. The levator ani muscle is seen with the inferior gluteal vessels lateral to it. The ligamentum teres within the fovea capitis of the right femur is visible.

4.9

1   Popliteus Tendon.
2   Anterior Cruciate Ligament.

3   Posterior Cruciate Ligament.
4   Medial Collateral Ligament.
5   Medial Tibial Spine.

Coronal MRI knee.

The groove on the lateral surface of the lateral femoral condyle where the popliteus tendon inserts is seen.

4.10
1   Stomach.
2   Spleen.
3   Portal Vein.
4   D2.
5   Urinary Bladder.

Coronal T2W MRI.

4.11
1   Pons.
2   Clivus.
3   **Posterior Arch of Atlas (C1).**
4   Anterior Longitudinal Ligament.
5   Interspinous Ligament.

Sagittal T2W MRI cervical spine.

In the '3 column' concept of the spine, used to assess radiological stability of spinal fractures:

> **Anterior Column:** Anterior longitudinal ligament and anterior half of vertebral body
> **Middle Column:** Posterior longitudinal ligament and posterior half of vertebral body
> **Posterior Column:** Ligamentum flavum, facet joints, posterior elements and interspinous ligaments.

4.12
1   1st Thoracic Vertebra (Right Aspect).
2   Head of Right Clavicle.
3   Acromion of Right Scapula.
4   Coracoid Process of Right Scapula.
5   Right Infraspinatus Muscle.

Lateral shoulder radiograph – 'Y' view.

Unlabelled, but convention dictates this is the right shoulder. This view adds further information when humeral head dislocation is suspected. The coracoid is the most anterior part of the scapula and should be used for orientation. This indicates that posterior to the scapula on the lateral view is the infraspinatus fossa where this muscle is found. The cradle of the 'Y' forms the supraspinatus fossa, and anterior to the scapula, between scapula and ribcage lies the subscapularis fossa.

4.13
1 **Right Infraorbital Canal**.
2 **Left Nasolacriminal Duct**.
3 Right Temporalis Muscle.
4 Right Pharyngeal Recess (Fossa of Rosenmüller).
5 Right Styloid Process.

Axial CT facial bones.

The pharyngeal recess, important in diagnosis of nasopharyngeal malignancy is seen, with the torus tubarius anterior to it. Obliteration or asymmetry of the recess, in the correct clinical setting, may indicate a soft tissue lesion or lymphadenopathy at this site.

4.14
1 Soleus Muscle.
2 Flexor Hallucis Longus Muscle.
3 Tendon of Tibialis Anterior.
4 Tendon of Flexor Hallucis Longus.
5 Flexor Digitorum Brevis Muscle.

Sagittal MRI ankle.

The sinus tarsi, tendoachilles and plantar fascia are also demonstrated. Within the sinus tarsi lies the talocalcaneal ligament.

4.15
1 Right Ischial Tuberosity.
2 Right Corpus Cavernosum.
3 Levator Ani Muscle.
4 Left Quadratus Femoris Muscle.
5 Left Sartorius Muscle.

Axial T1W MRI male pelvis.

The adductors and anterior thigh muscles are well seen. Adjacent to the ischial tuberosity lies the sciatic nerve. The relationship between levator ani and the ischioanal fossa is again demonstrated.

4.16
1 Right Forceps Minor.
2 Right External Capsule.
3 Right Aspect of Thalamus.
4 Trigone of Right Lateral Ventricle.
5 Left Lenticulostriate Arteries, Branches of the Left MCA.

Axial FLAIR MRI brain.

Demonstrated as a FLAIR sequence by the high signal grey matter, low signal white matter and lack of signal from CSF. The signal from fluid has been nulled due to the timing of the MR pulses. Forceps minor is the extension of the genu of the corpus callosum into each frontal lobe.

4.17
1   **Right Ventricle.**
2   **Gastroduodenal Artery.**
3   Gallbladder.
4   Stomach.
5   L1 Vertebra.

Coronal CT angiogram.

The head of the pancreas within the 'C' loop of duodenum is seen. The gallbladder is a fluid density structure, measuring approximately 0HU, and with a thin wall.

4.18
1   Right CN VII.
2   Right Vestibule.
3   Left CN VIII.
4   Right Middle Cerebellar Peduncle.
5   4th Ventricle.

Axial MRI IAM.

Meckel's cave can be seen bilaterally. This is an extension of the subarachnoid space and therefore, containing CSF, returns high signal on this study. It contains the trigeminal ganglion:

   V1: Ophthalmic Division – passes through superior orbital fissure
   V2: Maxillary Division – passes through foramen rotundum
   V3: Mandibular Division – passes through foramen ovale.

4.19
1   Left Rectus Femoris Muscle.
2   Left Adductor Longus Muscle.
3   Left Gracilis Muscle.
4   Right Iliotibial Tract.
5   Left Biceps Femoris Muscle.

Axial T1W MRI upper thigh.

The iliotibial tract is a fibrous band running from the ilium to the lateral femoral condyle. It serves as a point of attachment for various muscles. Gluteus maximus can be identified posteriorly due to the orientation of its fibres. The femoral vessels and sciatic nerve can also be identified.

4.20
1   Lateral Ventricle.
2   Mammillary Body.
3   4th Ventricle.
4   Straight Sinus.
5   Aqueduct of Sylvius.

Sagittal MRI brain.

The straight sinus is seen overlying the tentorium cerebelli.

The superior cerebellar peduncle extends into the quadrigeminal plate, with the quadrigeminal cistern posterior to this.

Exam 5

5.1

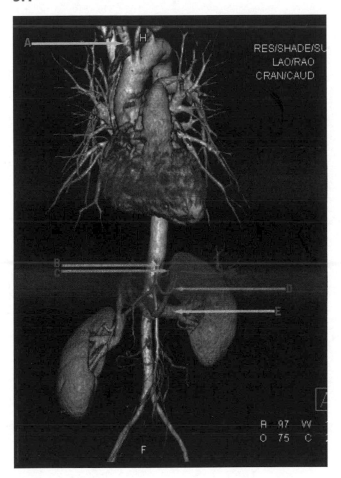

Answer the following questions.

1 Name structure 'A'.
2 Name structure 'B'.
3 Name structure 'C'.
4 Name structure 'D'.
5 Name structure 'E'.

5.2

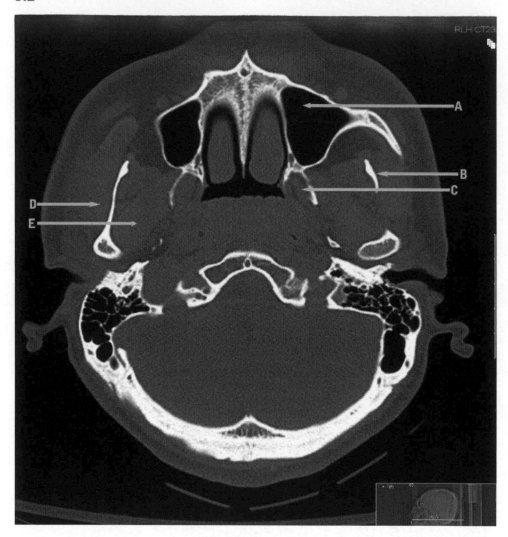

Answer the following questions.

1   Name structure 'A'.
2   Name structure 'B'.
3   Name structure 'C'.
4   Name structure 'D'.
5   Name structure 'E'.

5.3

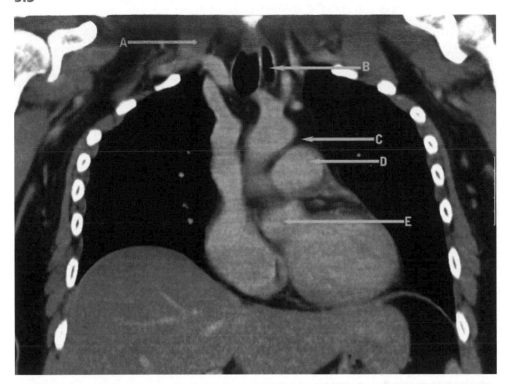

Answer the following questions.

1   Name structure 'A'.
2   Name structure 'B'.
3   Name structure 'C'.
4   Name structure 'D'.
5   Name structure 'E'.

5.4

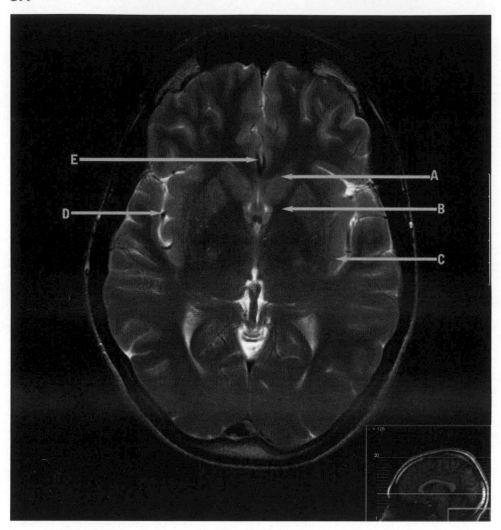

Answer the following questions.

1   Name structure 'A'.
2   Name structure 'B'.
3   Name structure 'C'.
4   Name structure 'D'.
5   Name structure 'E'.

5.5

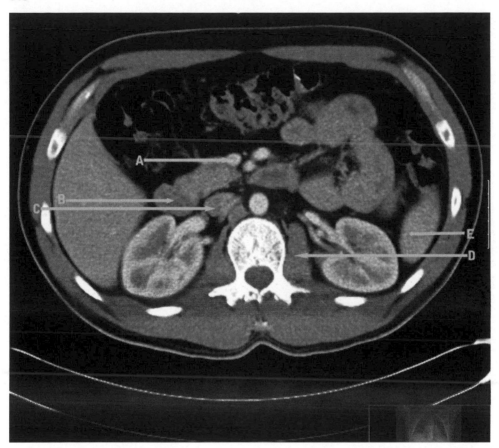

Answer the following questions.

1   Name structure 'A'.
2   Name structure 'B'.
3   Name structure 'C'.
4   Name structure 'D'.
5   Name structure 'E'.

5.6

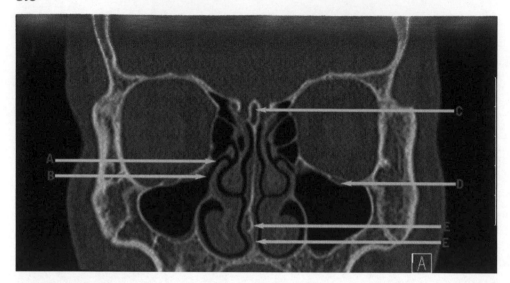

Answer the following questions.

1   Name structure 'A'.
2   Name structure 'B'.
3   Name structure 'C'.
4   The nerve found in 'D' originates from which cranial nerve?
5   Name structure 'E'.

5.7

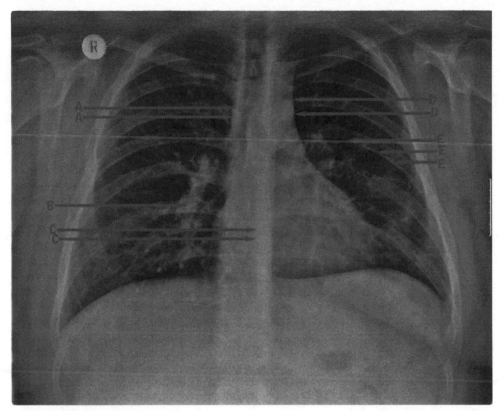

Answer the following questions.

1   Name structure 'A'.
2   Name structure 'B'.
3   Name structure 'C'.
4   Name structure 'D'.
5   Name structure 'E'.

5.8

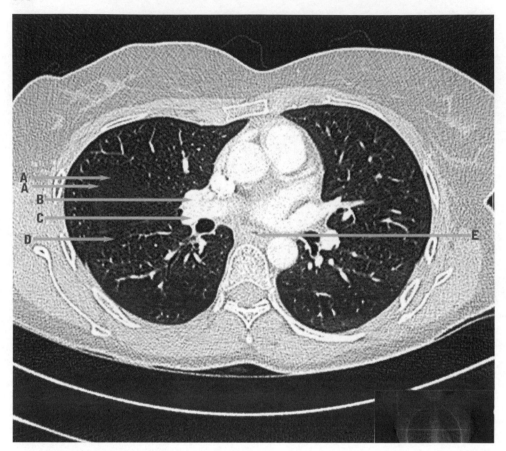

Answer the following questions.

1   Name structure 'A'.
2   Name structure 'B'.
3   Name structure 'C'.
4   Name structure 'D'.
5   Name structure 'E'.

5.9

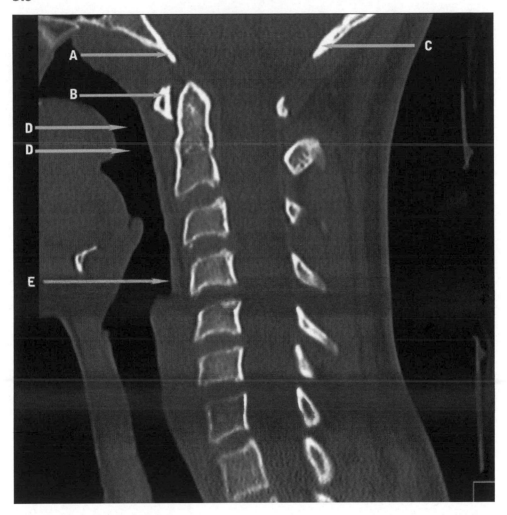

Answer the following questions.

1 Name structure 'A'.
2 Name structure 'B'.
3 Name structure 'C'.
4 Name structure 'D'.
5 What is the normal maximum width of structure 'E'?

5.10

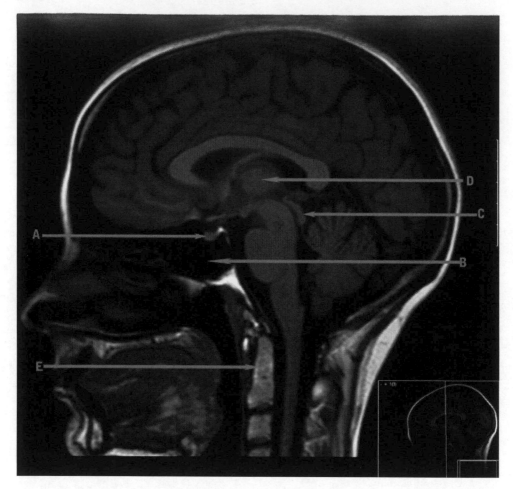

Answer the following questions.

1 Name structure 'A'.
2 Where does structure 'B' drain?
3 Name structure 'C'.
4 Name structure 'D'.
5 Name structure 'E'.

5.11

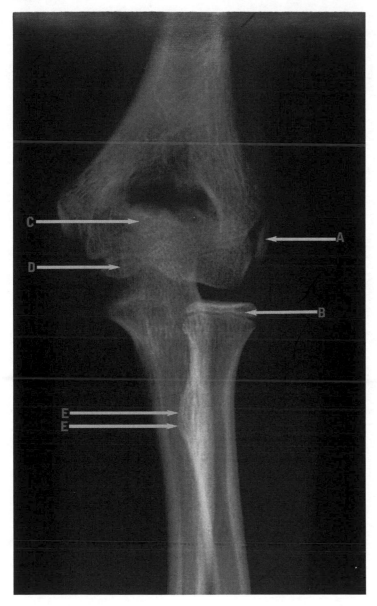

Answer the following questions.

1   Name structure 'A'.
2   Name structure 'B'.
3   Name structure 'C'.
4   Name structure 'D'.
5   Name structure 'E'.

5.12

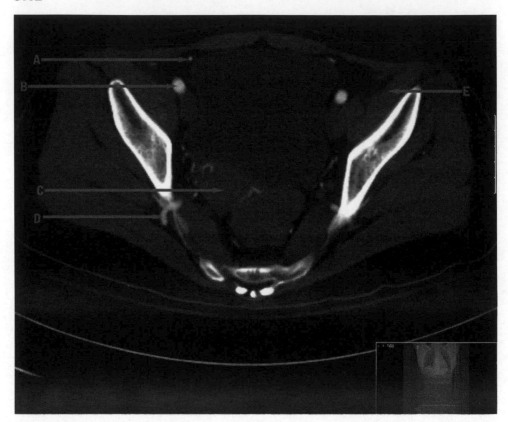

Answer the following questions.

1   Name structure 'A'.
2   Name structure 'B'.
3   Name structure 'C'.
4   Name structure 'D'.
5   Name structure 'E'.

5.13

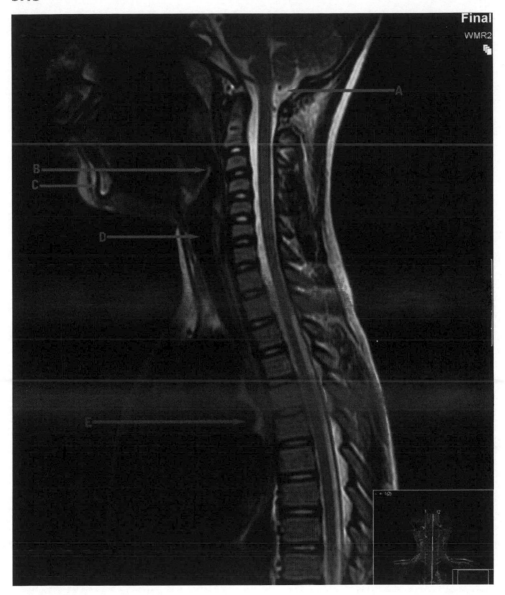

Answer the following questions.

1 Name structure 'A'.
2 Name structure 'B'.
3 Name structure 'C'.
4 Name structure 'D'.
5 Name structure 'E'.

5.14

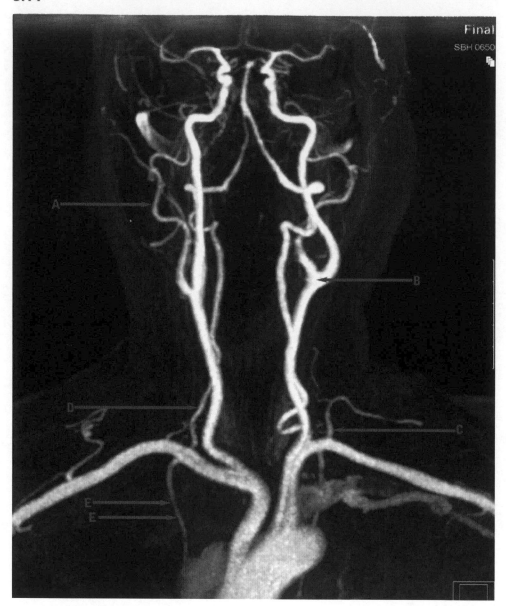

Answer the following questions.

1 Name structure 'A'.
2 Name structure 'B'.
3 Name structure 'C'.
4 Name structure 'D'.
5 Name structure 'E'.

5.15

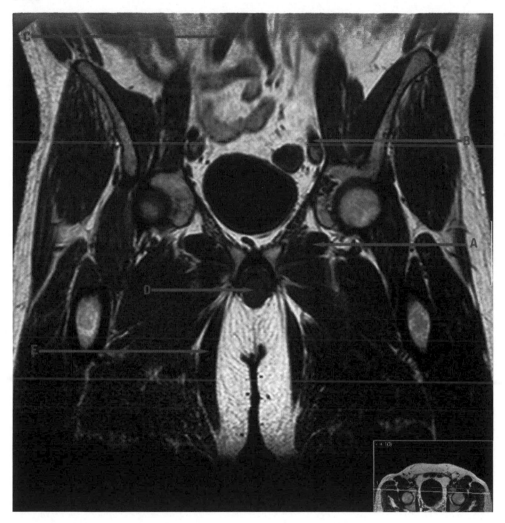

Answer the following questions.

1 Name structure 'A'.
2 Name structure 'B'.
3 Name structure 'C'.
4 Name structure 'D'.
5 Name structure 'E'.

5.16

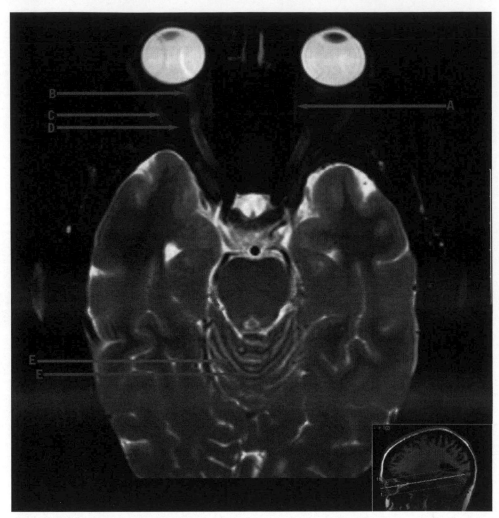

Answer the following questions.

1   Name structure 'A'.
2   Name structure 'B'.
3   Name structure 'C'.
4   Name structure 'D'.
5   Name structure 'E'.

5.17

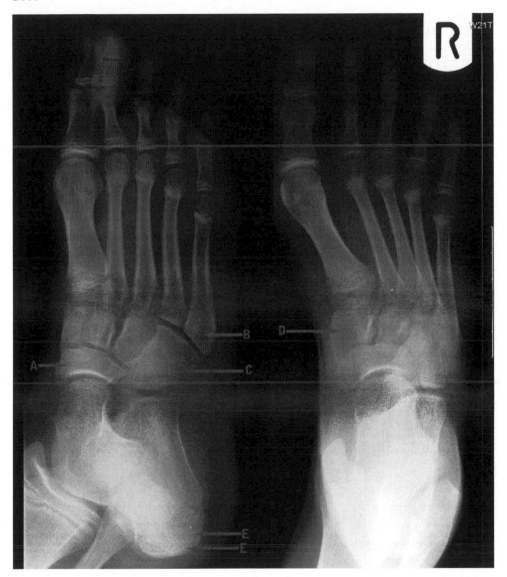

Answer the following questions.

1 Name structure 'A'.
2 Name structure 'B'.
3 Name structure 'C'.
4 Name structure 'D'.
5 Name structure 'E'.

5.18

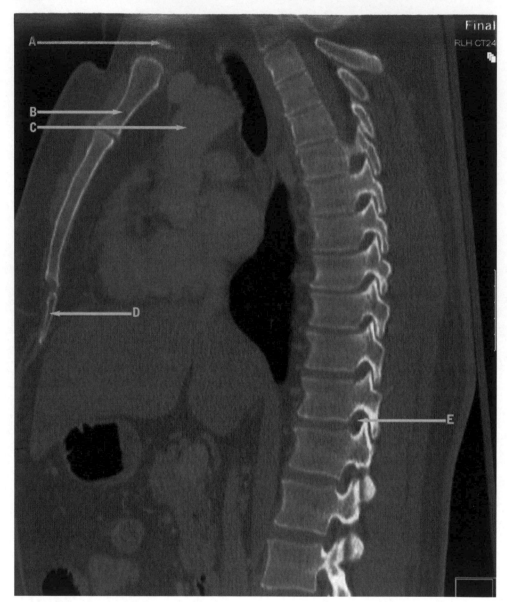

Answer the following questions.

1   Name structure 'A'.
2   Name structure 'B'.
3   Name structure 'C'.
4   Name structure 'D'.
5   Name structure 'E'.

5.19

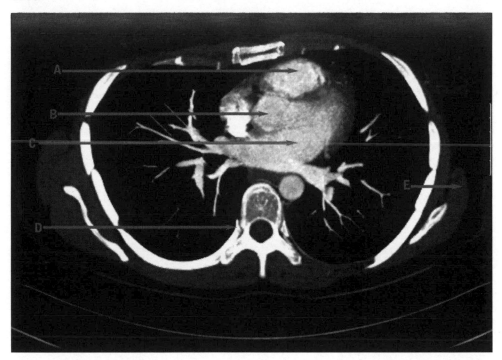

Answer the following questions.

1 Name structure 'A'.
2 Name structure 'B'.
3 Name structure 'C'.
4 Name structure 'D'.
5 Name structure 'E'.

5.20

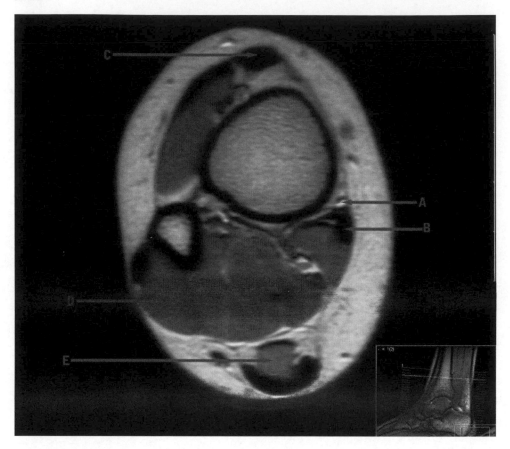

Answer the following questions.

1   Name structure 'A'.
2   Name structure 'B'.
3   Name structure 'C'.
4   Name structure 'D'.
5   Name structure 'E'.

Answers

5.1
1 Brachiocephalic Trunk.
2 Coeliac Axis.
3 Left Gastric Artery.
4 Splenic Artery.
5 Left Renal Vein.

Volume rendered reformat CT aortic angiogram.

5.2
1 Left Maxillary Antrum.
2 Coronoid Process of Left Mandible.
3 Left Medial Pterygoid Muscle.
4 **Right Masseter Muscle.**
5 Right Lateral Pterygoid Muscle.

Axial CT base of skull – bone windows.

The pterygoid plates and pterygoid fossae are seen. Anterior to this lies the pterygomaxillary fissure, a passage between the middle cranial fossa and infratemporal fossa. As such it is important in the spread of infection.

5.3
1 Right Sternocleidomastoid Muscle.
2 Oesophagus.
3 Aortopulmonary Window.
4 Pulmonary Trunk.
5 Aortic Root.

Coronal contrast enhanced CT chest.

5.4
1 Head of Left Caudate Nucleus.
2 Genu of Left Internal Capsule.
3 Left Claustrum.
4 Branch of Right Middle Cerebral Artery in Sylvian Fissure.
5 Right Anterior Cerebral Artery.

Axial T2W MRI brain.

The basal ganglia structures are demonstrated.

Vascular structures are seen as signal voids.

5.5
1   Superior Mesenteric Vein.
2   D2.
3   Inferior Vena Cava.
4   Left Psoas Muscle.
5   Spleen.

Axial contrast enhanced CT abdomen.

The small calibre, central small bowel loops can be differentiated from the outer, large calibre gas containing large bowel.

5.6
1   Right Infundibulum of Osteomeatal Unit.
2   Osteum of Right Osteomeatal Unit.
3   Crista Galli.
4   Left Trigeminal Nerve via Maxillary Division.
5   Vomer.

Coronal CT paranasal sinuses.

The OMU is demonstrated. The orbital floor and uncinate process of the ethmoid bone form the meatus and infundibulum through which secretions in the maxillary antra drain into the middle meatus, via the hiatus semilunaris.

5.7
1   Right Paratracheal Stripe.
2   Right Basal Pulmonary Artery.
3   Azygooesophageal Line.
4   Left Sided Superior Vena Cava.
5   Inferior Border of Posterior Left 7th Rib.

Frontal chest radiograph.

The azygooesophageal line is formed by the air/soft tissue interface between the right lung and azygos vein. It is altered in pathology arising from the middle or posterior mediastinum.

The normal paratracheal stripe should not measure more than 2–3mm.

5.8
1   Horizontal Fissure.
2   Right Superior Pulmonary Vein.
3   Right Pulmonary Artery.
4   Oblique Fissure of Right Lung.
5   Oesophagus.

HRCT chest.

The fissures are seen as areas where there is a paucity of lung markings. It can be seen that the right middle lobe abuts the right heart border, hence the loss of this silhouette in middle lobe pathology.

5.9
1   Clivus.
2   **Anterior Arch** of **Atlas (C1).**
3   Occipital Bone.
4   Oropharynx.
5   7mm at C3/4.

Sagittal CT cervical spine.

The width of the prevertebral soft tissues varies with the vertebral level. An accepted measurement for the upper limit of normal is 7mm at C3/4 and 21mm at C7. These measurements were previously made with lateral plain radiographs. Sagittal midline reformatted images now allow greater accuracy, and 18mm has been suggested as the upper limit of normal for soft tissues at C7. Widening may suggest ligamentous injury, haematoma or in non trauma cases, malignancy or abscess.

5.10
1   Anterior Pituitary Gland.
2   Sphenoethmoidal Recess.
3   Quadrigeminal Plate of Midbrain.
4   Thalamus.
5   Odontoid Peg of C2.

Sagittal MRI brain.

5.11
1   Centre for Lateral Epicondyle.
2   Centre for Radial Head.
3   Centre for Olecranon.
4   Centre for Trochlea.
5   Radial Tuberosity.

Anteroposterior paediatric elbow radiograph.

This child would be approximately 12–14 years old.

CRITOL
Capitulum
Radial Head
Internal (Medial) Epicondyle
Trochlea
Olecranon
Lateral Epicondyle.

5.12
1   Right Inferior Epigastric Artery.
2   Right External Iliac Artery.
3   Uterus.
4   Right Superior Gluteal Artery.
5   Left Iliopsoas Muscle.

Axial CT angiogram female pelvis.

The paired inferior epigastric artery and vein are visible. The inferior epigastric arteries anastomose with the superior epigastric artery which is a continuation of the internal thoracic artery. Iliopsoas is seen as it progresses laterally towards its insertion on the lesser trochanter.

5.13
1   Cisterna Magna.
2   Epiglottis.
3   Mandible.
4   Trachea.
5   Right Pulmonary Artery.

Sagittal MRI cervical spine.

5.14
1   Right External Carotid Artery.
2   Left Carotid Bulb.
3   Left Thyrocervical Trunk.
4   **Right Vertebral Artery.**
5   Right Internal Thoracic Artery.

Reformatted MR angiogram.

The branches of the external carotid artery are:

> **Superior thyroid artery**
> **Ascending pharyngeal artery**
> **L**ingual artery
> **F**acial artery
> **O**ccipital artery
> **P**osterior auricular artery.

Terminal branches:

> **M**axillary artery
> **S**uperficial temporal artery.

5.15
1   Left Pectineus Muscle.
2   Left External Iliac Artery.
3   Right Common Iliac Artery.
4   Bulb of Penis.
5   Right Gracilis Muscle.

Coronal MRI male pelvis.

5.16
1   Left Medial Rectus Muscle.
2   Right Optic Nerve.

3   Right Lateral Rectus Muscle.
4   Retro-orbital Fat of Right Eye.
5   Cerebellar Vermis.

Axial T2W MRI orbits.

The globes are high signal due to their fluid content. The globe and retro-orbital fat are rarely sites of metastatic spread and should be a review area in routine head imaging.

5.17

1   Right Navicular Bone.
2   Base of Right 5th Metatarsal Bone.
3   Right Cuboid Bone.
4   Right Medial Cunieform Bone.
5   Right Calcaneal Tuberosity.

Dorsoplantar and oblique foot radiographs.

The alignment of the midfoot can be seen, this normal appearance is lost in Lisfranc ligament injuries.

5.18

1   Head of Clavicle.
2   Manubrium of Sternum.
3   Ascending Aorta.
4   Xiphisternum.
5   **Intervertebral Foramen.**

Sagittal CT thoracolumbar spine – bone windows.

The intervertebral foramina are demonstrated. They have a keyhole appearance on sagittal images. The exiting nerve roots are as follows:

C1–7 – the exiting nerve root is that of the lower numbered vertebra, i.e. C6 root exits at C5/6
C7–T1 – C8 exits at this level
T1 onwards – the exiting nerve root is that of the higher vertebra, i.e. L4 root at L4/5.

5.19

1   Right Ventricle.
2   Aortic Root.
3   Left Atrium.
4   Head of Right Rib.
5   Left Latissimus Dorsi Muscle.

Axial CTPA maximum intensity projection (MIP).

The posterior position of the left atrium, and its ability to simulate a posterior mediastinal mass when enlarged, is demonstrated. Alteration of the azygooesophageal line is one manifestation. The left ventricle is differentiated from the right by its bulkier myocardium. Note the papillary muscles within the left ventricle.

5.20
1   Long Saphenous Vein.
2   Tendon of Tibialis Posterior.
3   Tendon of Tibialis Anterior.
4   Peroneus Brevis Muscle.
5   Soleus Muscle.

Axial MRI lower limb.

Although variable in their course, the following is useful in identifying the tendons and muscles of the lower limb.

From medial to lateral posterior to the medial malleolus:

Tom: Tibialis Posterior
Dick: Flexor Digitorum Longus
Harry: Flexor Hallucis Longus.

From medial to lateral, anterior to the medial malleolus:

Tom: Tibialis Anterior
Harry: Extensor Hallucis Longus
Dick: Extensor Digitorum.

Exam 6

6.1

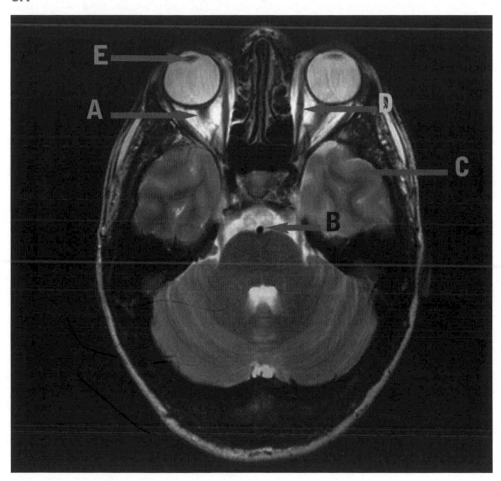

Answer the following questions.

1   Name structure 'A'.
2   Name structure 'B'.
3   Name structure 'C'.
4   Name structure 'D'.
5   Name structure 'E'.

6.2

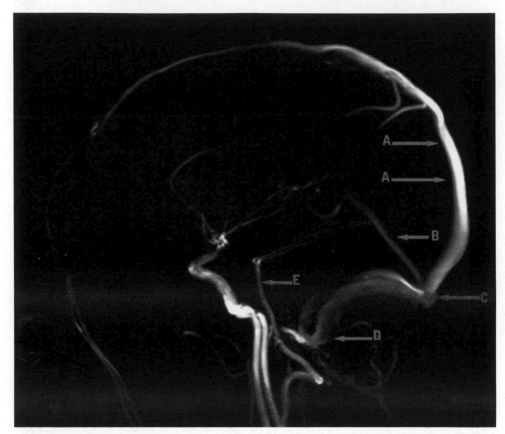

Answer the following questions.

1   Name structure 'A'.
2   Name structure 'B'.
3   Name structure 'C'.
4   Name structure 'D'.
5   Name structure 'E'.

6.3

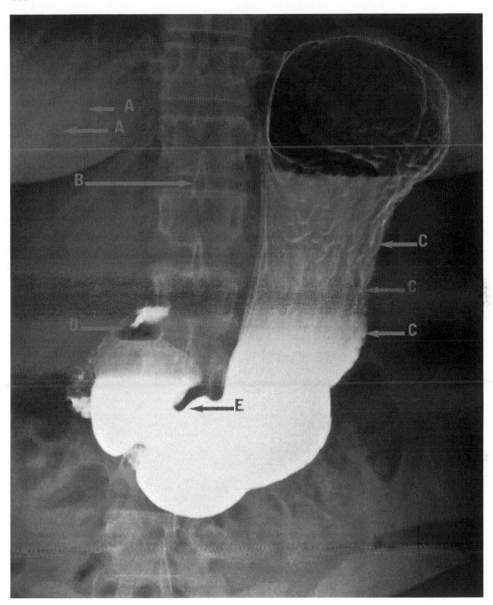

Answer the following questions.

1   Name structure 'A'.
2   Name structure 'B'.
3   Name structure 'C'.
4   Name structure 'D'.
5   Name structure 'E'.

6.4

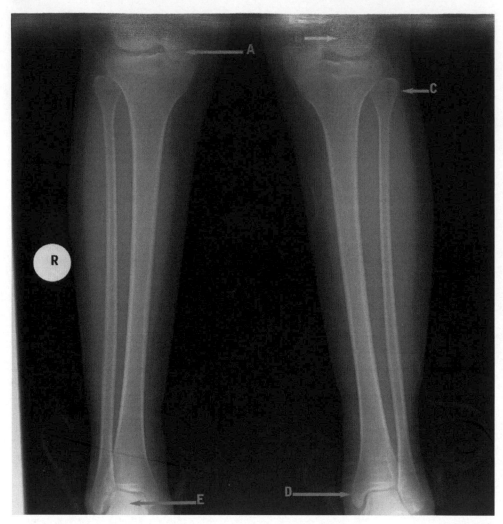

Answer the following questions.

1   Name structure 'A'.
2   Name structure 'B'.
3   Name structure 'C'.
4   Name structure 'D'.
5   Name structure 'E'.

6.5

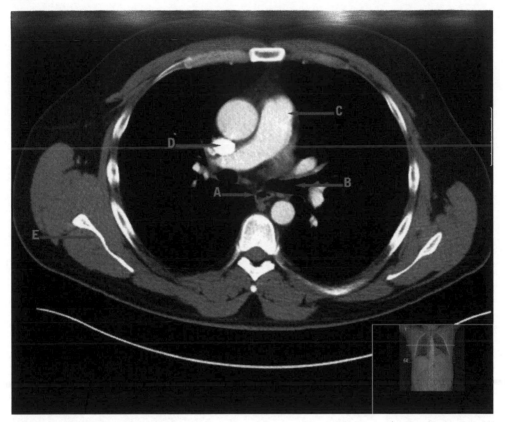

Answer the following questions.

1 Name structure 'A'.
2 Name structure 'B'.
3 Name structure 'C'.
4 Name structure 'D'.
5 Name structure 'E'.

6.6

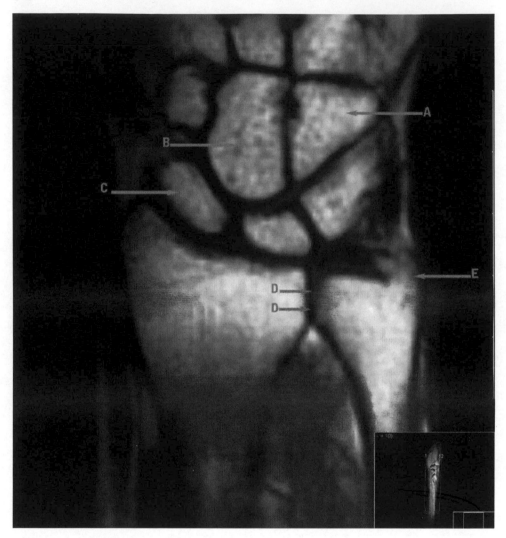

Answer the following questions.

1 Name structure 'A'.
2 Name structure 'B'.
3 Name structure 'C'.
4 Name structure 'D'.
5 Name structure 'E'.

6.7

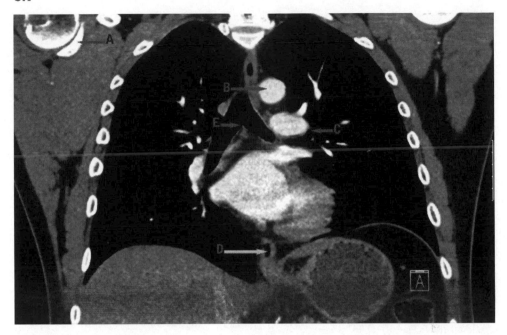

Answer the following questions.

1 Name structure 'A'.
2 **Name structure 'B'.**
3 **Name structure 'C'.**
4 Name structure 'D'.
5 Name structure 'E'.

6.8

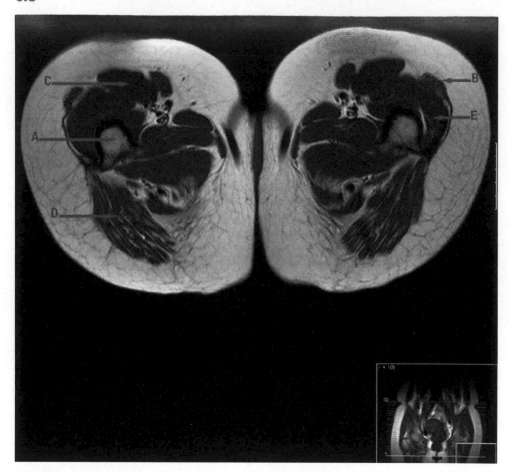

Answer the following questions.

1 Name structure 'A'.
2 Name structure 'B'.
3 Name structure 'C'.
4 Name structure 'D'.
5 Name structure 'E'.

6.9

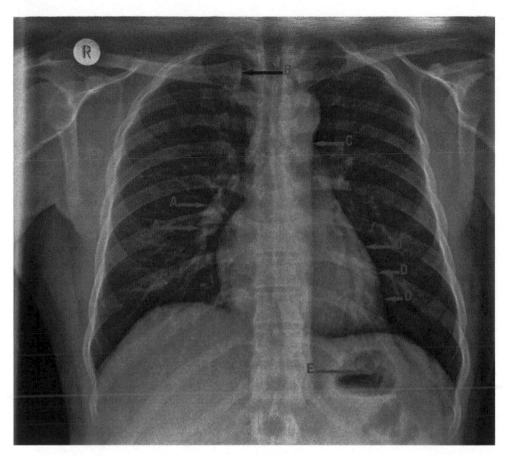

Answer the following questions.

1   Name structure 'A'.
2   Name structure 'B'.
3   Name structure 'C'.
4   Name structure 'D'.
5   Name structure 'E'.

6.10

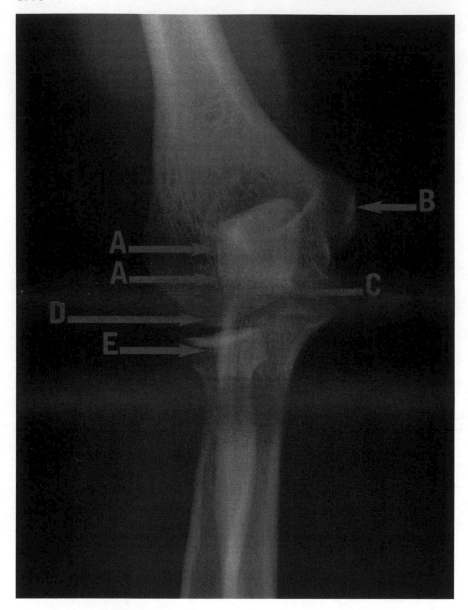

Answer the following questions.

1   Name structure 'A'.
2   Name structure 'B'.
3   Name structure 'C'.
4   Name structure 'D'.
5   Name structure 'E'.

6.11

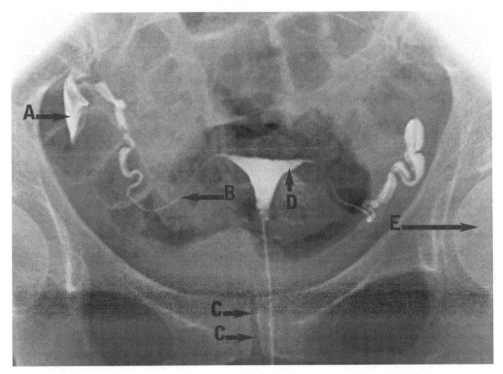

Answer the following questions.

1 Where is the contrast seen at 'A'?
2 Name structure 'B'.
3 Name structure 'C'.
4 Name structure 'D'.
5 Name structure 'E'.

6.12

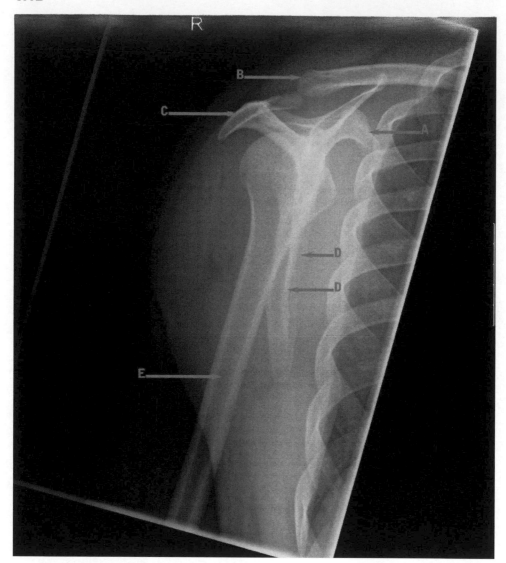

Answer the following questions.

1 Name structure 'A'.
2 Name structure 'B'.
3 Name structure 'C'.
4 Name structure 'D'.
5 Name structure 'E'.

6.13

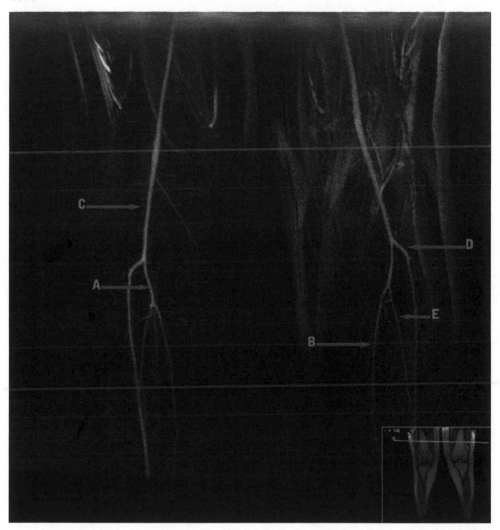

Answer the following questions.

1   Name structure 'A'.
2   Name structure 'B'.
3   Name structure 'C'.
4   Name structure 'D'.
5   Name structure 'E'.

6.14

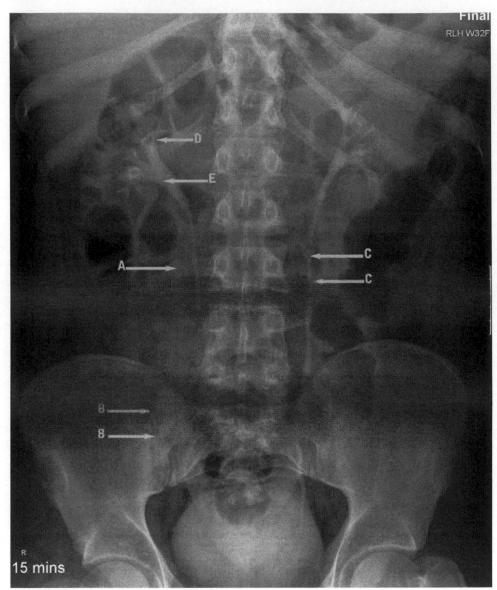

Answer the following questions.

1   Name structure 'A'.
2   Name structure 'B'.
3   Name structure 'C'.
4   Name structure 'D'.
5   Name structure 'E'.

6.15

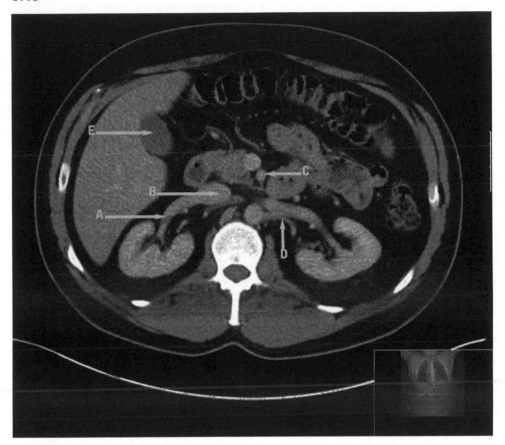

Answer the following questions.

1 Name structure 'A'.
2 Name structure 'B'.
3 Name structure 'C'.
4 Name structure 'D'.
5 Name structure 'E'.

6.16

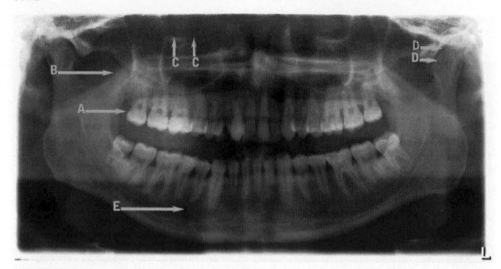

Answer the following questions.

1   Name structure 'A'.
2   Name structure 'B'.
3   Name structure 'C'.
4   Name structure 'D'.
5   Name structure 'E'.

6.17

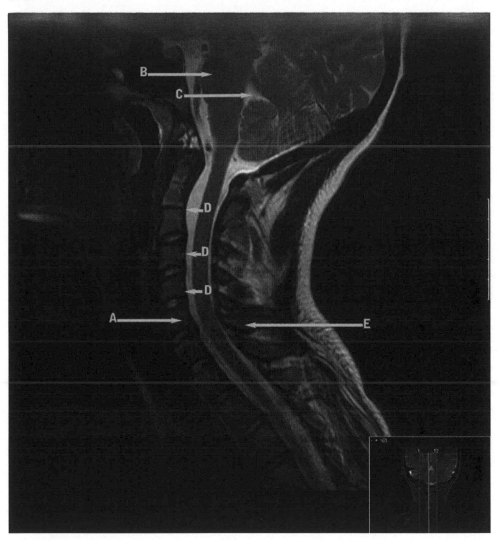

Answer the following questions.

1   Name structure 'A'.
2   Name structure 'B'.
3   Name structure 'C'.
4   Name structure 'D'.
5   Name structure 'E'.

6.18

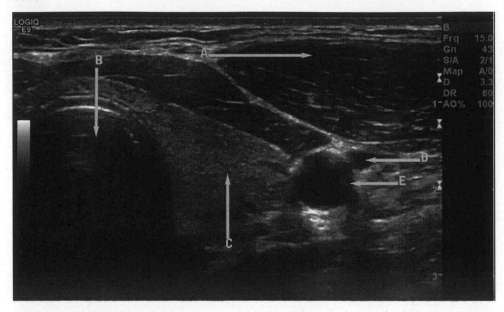

Answer the following questions.

1   Name structure 'A'.
2   Name structure 'B'.
3   Name structure 'C'.
4   **Name structure 'D'.**
5   Name structure 'E'.

6.19

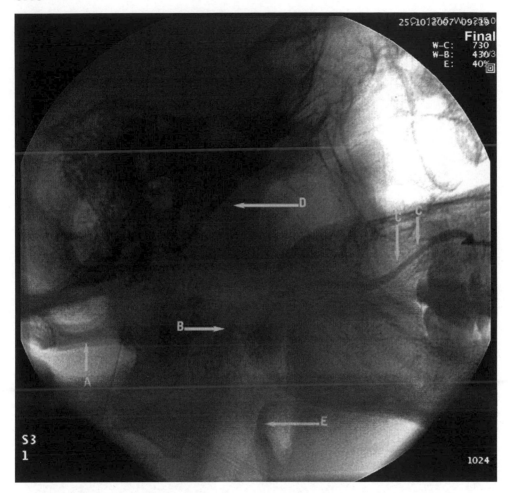

Answer the following questions.

1   Name structure 'A'.
2   Name structure 'B'.
3   Name structure 'C'.
4   Name structure 'D'.
5   Name structure 'E'.

6.20

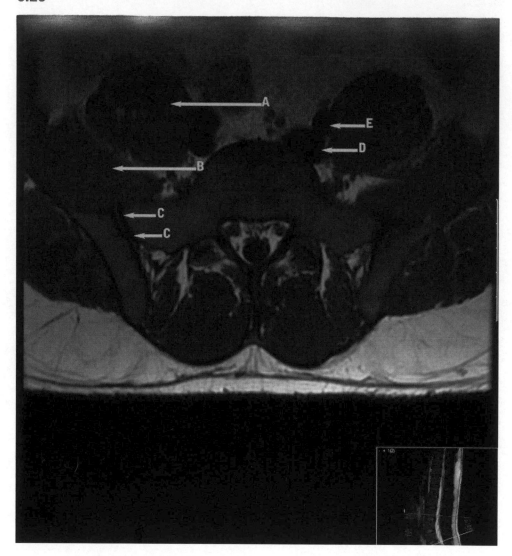

Answer the following questions.

1 Name structure 'A'.
2 Name structure 'B'.
3 Name structure 'C'.
4 Name structure 'D'.
5 Name structure 'E'.

Answers

6.1
1 Right Optic Nerve.
2 Basilar Artery.
3 Left Temporal Lobe.
4 Left Medial Rectus Muscle.
5 Lens of Right Eye.

Axial T2W MRI at level of pons.

The pons is continuous with the midbrain above and the medulla oblongata below. Present in the pons are several cranial nerve nuclei: the motor nucleus and a sensory nucleus of the trigeminal nerve (CNV), abducens nucleus (CNVI), facial nerve nucleus (CNVII) and the vestibulocochlear nuclei (CNVIII).

6.2
1 Superior Sagittal Sinus.
2 Straight Sinus.
3 Confluence of Venous Sinuses (Torcular Herophili).
4 Sigmoid Sinus.
5 Basilar Artery.

MRI veno/arteriogram.

On this image the venous sinuses as well as the arterial system is shown. MR angiography may be performed without intravenous contrast, instead utilising the flow characteristics of blood to form an image.

6.3
1 Right 11th Rib.
2 Spinous Process of T12.
3 Greater Curve of Stomach.
4 Duodenal Cap.
5 Pylorus.

Double contrast barium study of stomach.

6.4
1 Medial Condyle of Right Femur.
2 Left Patella.
3 Left Fibula Head.
4 Left Medial Malleolus (of Tibia).
5 Right Talus.

AP radiograph of both lower legs.

This question illustrates the importance of mentioning the laterality of a structure in your exam answers in order to gain all available marks.

6.5
1   Oesophagus.
2   Left Main Bronchus.
3   Pulmonary Trunk.
4   Superior Vena Cava.
5   Blade of Right Scapula.

Axial CTPA.

6.6
1   Hamate.
2   Capitate.
3   Scaphoid.
4   Distal Radio-Ulnar Joint.
5   Styloid Process of Ulna.

Coronal MRI wrist.

Though the view is limited, the distinctive shape of the distal radius is clear to see and therefore enables the carpals to be named.

6.7
1   Right Glenoid.
2   Arch of Aorta (Aortic Knuckle).
3   Left Superior Lobe bronchus.
4   Oesophagus.
5   Carina.

Coronal contrast enhanced CT chest.

6.8
1   Right Femoral Shaft.
2   Left Tensor Fasciae Latae Muscle.
3   Right Rectus Femoris Muscle.
4   Right Gluteus Maximus Muscle.
5   Left Vastus Lateralis Muscle.

Axial MRI thigh.

The thigh is divided into three fascial compartments by fibrous septa, each supplied by a different nerve. They are: **medial** (adductors, obturator nerve), **anterior** (quadriceps, sartorius, femoral nerve) and **posterior** (hamstring muscles, sciatic nerve).

6.9
1   Right Inferior Lobe Pulmonary Artery.
2   Head of Right Clavicle.
3   Aorto-Pulmonary Window.

4   Border of Left Ventricle.

5   Gas in Fundus of Stomach.

PA chest radiograph.

The aortopulmonary window contains the ligamentum arteriosum, lymph nodes, recurrent laryngeal nerve and fat.

6.10

1   Olecranon.

2   Medial Epicondyle of Humerus.

3   Trochlea.

4   Capitulum.

5   Head of Radius.

AP radiograph of elbow.

6.11

1   Intraperitoneal Contrast.

2   Right Uterine Tube.

3   Pubic Symphysis.

4   Left Cornu of Uterus.

5   Left Head of Femur.

Hysterosalpingogram (HSG).

The catheter can be seen at the base of the uterine cavity. The contrast seen at 'A' is **termed 'free spill' and demonstrates patency of the right uterine (also termed fallopian) tube**.

6.12

1   Coracoid Process of Right Scapula.

2   Distal Right Clavicle.

3   Acromion Process of Right Scapula.

4   Blade of Right Scapula.

5   Diaphysis (Shaft) of Right Humerus.

Lateral radiograph of right shoulder (Y-view).

This view is useful for assessing the position of the humeral head relative to the glenoid. It enables dislocations to be classified into anterior or posterior and gives information on the position of fracture fragments.

6.13

1   Right Tibioperoneal Trunk.

2   Left Posterior Tibial Artery.

3   Right Popliteal Artery.

4   Left Anterior Tibial Artery.

5   Left Peroneal Artery.

Coronal MRI arteriogram lower limbs.

Just above arrow 'C', the joint line of the knee can be seen. The popliteal artery is a continuation of the superficial femoral artery. It extends from the adductor hiatus to the fibrous arch of soleus. Before its trifurcation, it gives off muscular and genicular branches which supply the muscles and support structures around the knee.

6.14
1   Right Transverse Process of L3.
2   Right Sacroiliac Joint.
3   Left Ureter.
4   Right Upper Pole Minor Calyx.
5   Right Renal Pelvis.

IVU excretory phase.

6.15
1   Right Renal Vein.
2   Inferior Vena Cava.
3   Superior Mesenteric Artery.
4   Left Renal Artery.
5   Gallbladder.

Axial CT abdomen.

The relationship between the superior mesenteric artery and vein (anterior to artery) can be seen. Also the usual appearance of the SMA is seen with its surrounding ring of fat. This is often lost in infiltrative disease. This image is taken at the transpyloric plane (L1/2).

6.16
1   Right Upper 3rd Molar.
2   Right Coronoid Process of Mandible.
3   Right Inferior Orbital Ridge.
4   Left Temporo-Mandibular Joint.
5   Right Mental Foramen.

Orthopantomogram (OPG).

This image is taken using a tomographic technique to give a panoramic representation of the mandible and dentition. The mental foramen transmits the mental nerve and vessels. The mental nerve is a branch of the inferior alveolar nerve. It provides sensation to the anterior chin and lower lip.

6.17
1   Vertebral Body of C6.
2   Pons.
3   4th Ventricle.
4   Posterior Longitudinal Ligament.
5   Spinous Process of C7.

Sagittal T2W MRI neck.

The CSF spaces appear bright on T2W MRI. Anterior to the vertebral bodies, the anterior longitudinal ligament can be seen. The **ligamentum flavum (yellow ligaments)** can be seen posterior to the epidural fat.

6.18
1   Left Sternocleidomastoid Muscle.
2   Trachea.
3   Left Lobe of Thyroid.
4   Left Internal Jugular Vein.
5   Left Common Carotid Artery.

Axial ultrasound of left lobe of thyroid.

6.19
1   Spinous Process of C1.
2   Secondary Parotid Ductules.
3   Parotid (Stenson's) Duct.
4   Condyle of Mandible.
5   Epiglottis.

Parotid sialogram.

The catheter can be seen at the opening of Stenson's duct. This lies on the mucous membrane of the cheek opposite the 2nd upper molar.

6.20
1   Right Psoas Muscle.
2   Right Iliacus Muscle.
3   Right Sacroiliac Joint.
4   Left Common Iliac Vein.
5   Left Common Iliac Artery.

Axial T2W MRI pelvis.

The image is taken at the pelvic brim, at which level the common iliac vessels bifurcate to form the internal and external iliacs.

Iliacus arises from the upper iliac fossa and inserts into the psoas tendon and the adjacent part of the femur below the lesser trochanter. Alongside the psoas it is a powerful flexor of the hip.

Exam 7

7.1

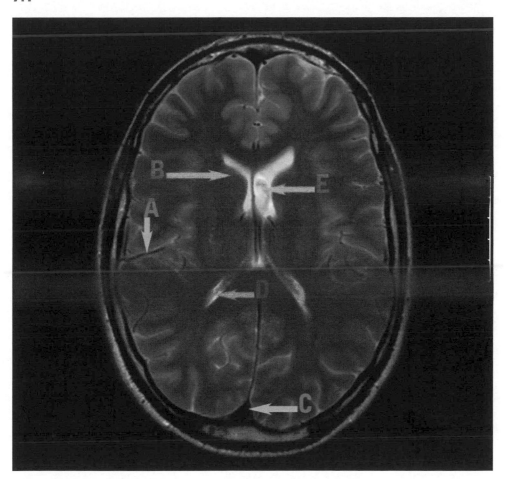

Answer the following questions.

1. Name structure 'A'.
2. Name structure 'B'.
3. Name structure 'C'.
4. Name structure 'D'.
5. Name structure 'E'.

7.2

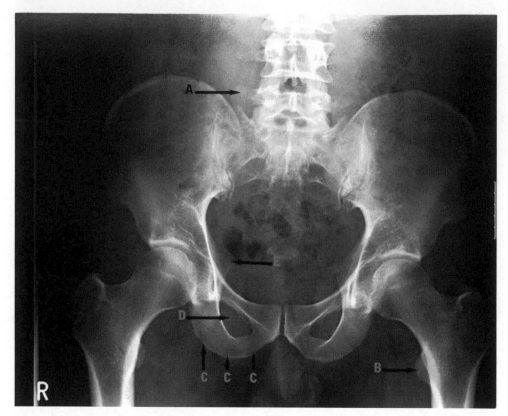

Answer the following questions.

1 Name structure 'A'.
2 Name structure 'B'.
3 Name structure 'C'.
4 What passes through foramen 'D'?
5 Name structure 'E'.

7.3

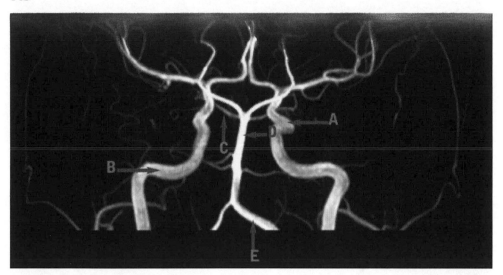

Answer the following questions.

1   Name structure 'A'.
2   Name structure 'B'.
3   Name structure 'C'.
4   Name structure 'D'.
5   Name structure 'E'.

7.4

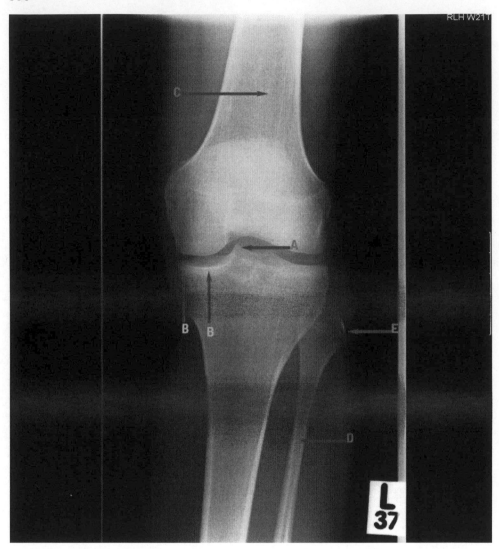

Answer the following questions.

1 What attaches at 'A'?
2 Name structure 'B'.
3 Name structure 'C'.
4 Name structure 'D'.
5 Name structure 'E'.

7.5

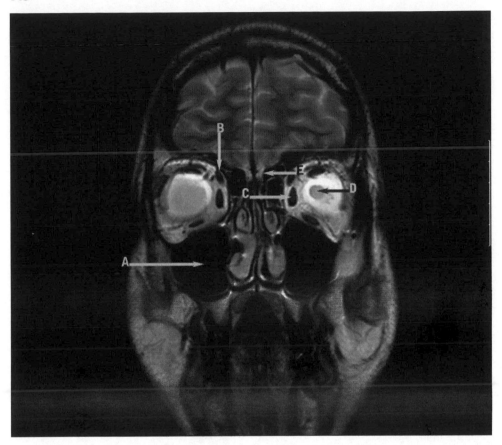

Answer the following questions.

1   Name structure 'A'.
2   What nerve innervates muscle 'B'?
3   Name structure 'C'.
4   Name structure 'D'.
5   Name structure 'E'.

7.6

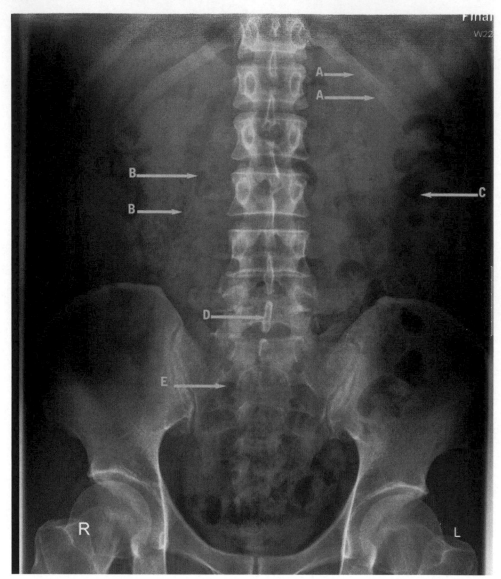

Answer the following questions.

1   Name structure 'A'.
2   Name structure 'B'.
3   Name structure 'C'.
4   Name structure 'D'.
5   Name structure 'E'.

7.7

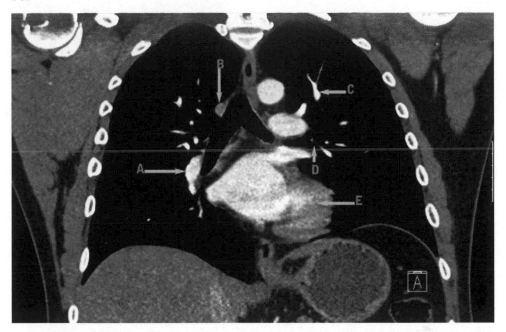

Answer the following questions.

1 Name structure 'A'.
2 Name structure 'B'.
3 Name structure 'C'.
4 Name structure 'D'.
5 Name structure 'E'.

7.8

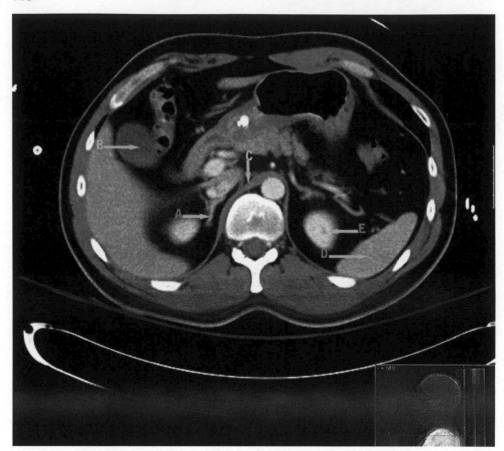

Answer the following questions.

1 Name structure 'A'.
2 Name structure 'B'.
3 Name structure 'C'.
4 Name structure 'D'.
5 Name structure 'E'.

7.9

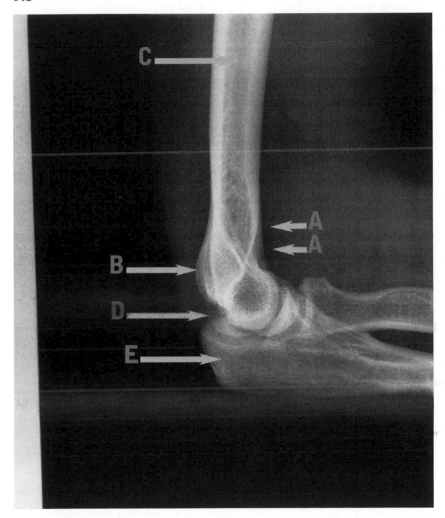

Answer the following questions.

1   Name structure 'A'.
2   Name structure 'B'.
3   Name structure 'C'.
4   Name structure 'D'.
5   Name structure 'E'.

7.10

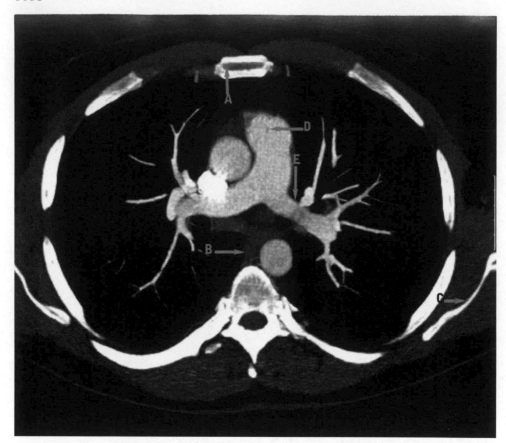

Answer the following questions.

1 Name structure 'A'.
2 Name structure 'B'.
3 Name structure 'C'.
4 Name structure 'D'.
5 Name structure 'E'.

7.11

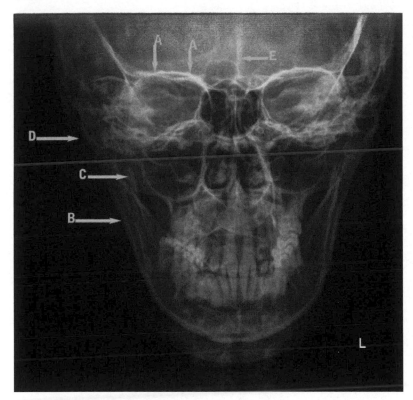

Answer the following questions.

1   Name structure 'A'.
2   Name structure 'B'.
3   Name structure 'C'.
4   Name structure 'D'.
5   Name structure 'E'.

7.12

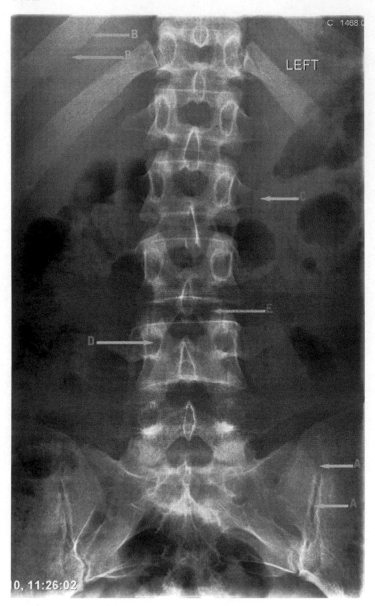

Answer the following questions.

1   Name structure 'A'.
2   Name structure 'B'.
3   Name structure 'C'.
4   Name structure 'D'.
5   Name structure 'E'.

7.13

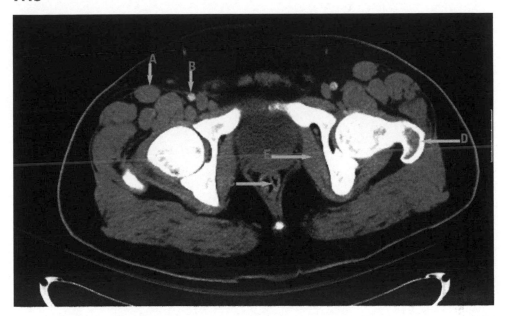

Answer the following questions.

1   Name structure 'A'.
2   Name structure 'B'.
3   Name structure 'C'.
4   **Name structure 'D'.**
5   Name structure 'E'.

7.14

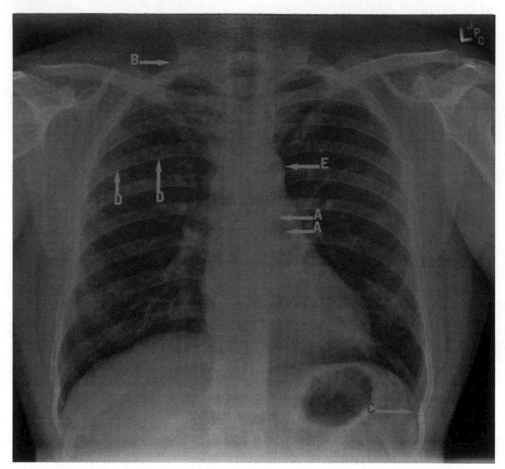

Answer the following questions.

1   Name structure 'A'.
2   Name structure 'B'.
3   Name structure 'C'.
4   Name structure 'D'.
5   Name structure 'E'.

7.15

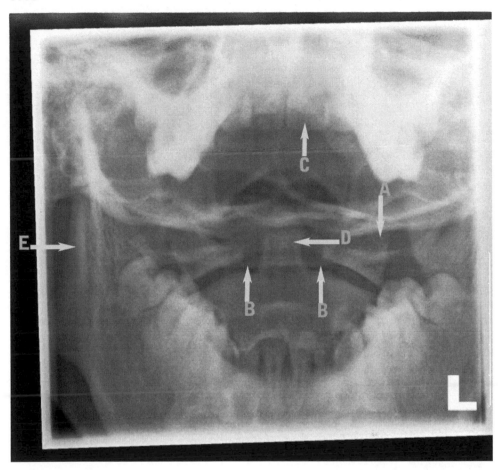

Answer the following questions.

1 Name structure 'A'.
2 Name structure 'B'.
3 Name structure 'C'.
4 Name structure 'D'.
5 Name structure 'E'.

7.16

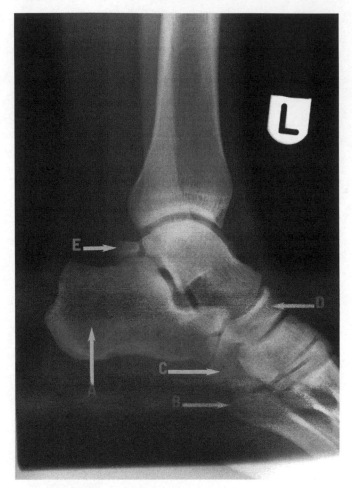

Answer the following questions.

1   Name structure 'A'.
2   Name structure 'B'.
3   Name structure 'C'.
4   Name structure 'D'.
5   What normal variant is seen at 'E'?

7.17

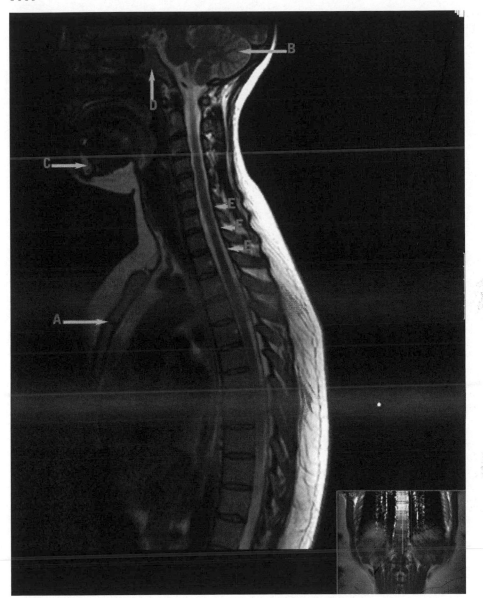

Answer the following questions.

1   Name structure 'A'.
2   Name structure 'B'.
3   Name structure 'C'.
4   Name structure 'D'.
5   Name structure 'E'.

7.18

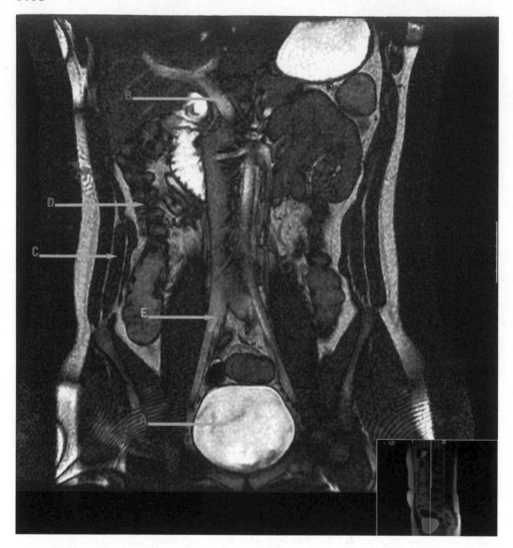

Answer the following questions.

1   Name structure 'A'.
2   Name structure 'B'.
3   Name structure 'C'.
4   Name structure 'D'.
5   Name structure 'E'.

7.19

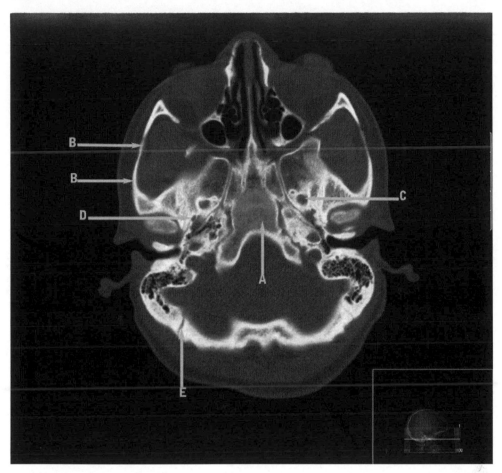

Answer the following questions.

1 Name structure 'A'.
2 Name structure 'B'.
3 Name structure 'C'.
4 Name structure 'D'.
5 Name structure 'E'.

7.20

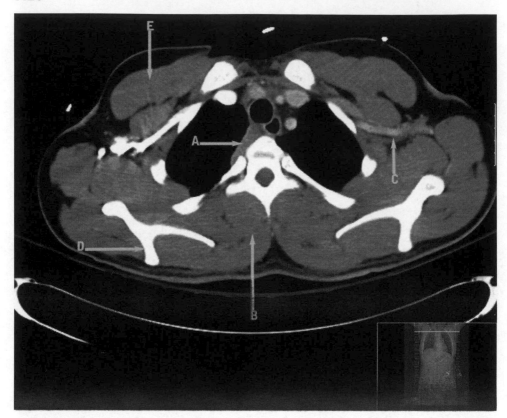

Answer the following questions.

1 Name structure 'A'.
2 Name structure 'B'.
3 Name structure 'C'.
4 Name structure 'D'.
5 Name structure 'E'.

Answers

7.1
1 Right Sylvian Fissure.
2 Head of Right Caudate Nucleus.
3 Superior Sagittal Sinus.
4 Posterior Horn of Right Lateral Ventricle.
5 Left Lateral Ventricle.

Axial T2W MRI.

The choroid plexus is found in the posterior body of the lateral ventricle and produces CSF.

7.2
1 Right Transverse Process of L5.
2 Left Lesser Trochanter.
3 Right Inferior Pubic Ramus.
4 Right Obturator Vessels and Nerve.
5 Right Ischial Tuberosity.

AP pelvis radiograph.

The obturator foramen appears large on imaging, however it is largely covered with the obturator membrane. It transmits the obturator vessels and nerve; the artery is a branch of the anterior division of the internal liac artery. The obturator nerve is a branch of the lumbar plexus, it supplies the adductor compartment of the thigh.

7.3
1 Cavernous Portion of Left Internal Carotid Artery.
2 Petrous Portion of Right Internal Carotid Artery.
3 Right Superior Cerebellar Artery.
4 Basilar Artery.
5 Left Vertebral Artery.

AP view 3-D MRA reformat.

7.4
1 Left Anterior Cruciate Ligament.
2 Left Medial Tibial Condyle.
3 Diaphysis of Left Femur.
4 Diaphysis of Left Fibula.
5 Head of Left Fibula.

AP radiograph left knee.

The ACL attaches to the anterior part of the tibial plateau between the attachments of the anterior horns of the medial and lateral menisci. This is just anterior to the medial intercondylar tubercle. Its femoral attachment is on the posteromedial aspect of the lateral condyle.

The PCL has a broader attachment on the posterior intecondylar area and ascends to the anterolateral aspect of the medial femoral condyle.

7.5
1   Right Maxillary Sinus.
2   Right Cranial Nerve IV (Trochlear Nerve).
3   Left Medial Rectus Muscle.
4   Left Optic Nerve.
5   Left Olfactory Bulb.

Coronal MRI orbits.

The superior oblique is supplied by CN IV. The other muscles of the orbit are supplied by CN III (oculomotor) except lateral rectus which is supplied by CN VI (abducens).

7.6
1   Left 12th rib.
2   Right Psoas Shadow.
3   Gas in Descending Colon.
4   Spinous Process of L5.
5   Right Anterior Sacral Foramen.

AP abdominal radiograph.

The sacral foramina transmit the anterior and posterior rami of the sacral nerves.

7.7
1   Right Inferior Lobe Artery.
2   Azygous Vein.
3   Left Superior Lobe Artery.
4   Left Inferior Lobe Bronchus.
5   Left Ventricle.

Coronal contrast enhanced CT chest.

The relationship of the azygos vein to the right hilum is demonstrated. At the level of T4 it arches forward over the right lung hilum to enter the superior vena cava (SVC).

7.8
1   Medial Limb of Right Adrenal.
2   Gall Bladder.
3   Right Crus of Diaphragm.
4   Spleen.
5   Upper Pole of Left Kidney.

Axial contrast enhanced CT abdomen.

The relationship between the left and right crus of the diaphragm and the abdominal Aorta can be seen. The crura are strong tendons attached to the upper lumbar vertebrae.

Diaphragmatic openings:

> Aortic (T12) – aorta, azygos vein, thoracic duct
> Oesophageal (T10) – oesophagus
> Vena Caval (T8) – inferior vena cava.

7.9
1 Anterior Fat Pad.
2 Medial Epicondyle.
3 Diaphysis of Humerus.
4 Trochlea.
5 Olecranon.

Lateral radiograph adult Elbow.

No side is indicated therefore laterality cannot be ascertained. The anterior fat pad is normally barely visible in a normal individual, the posterior pad should not be seen at all. Visible posterior fat pad or elevation of the anterior pad post injury represent intra-articular haemorrhage or effusion and careful scrutiny is needed to identify subtle fractures.

7.10
1 Sternum.
2 Azygos Vein.
3 Blade of Left Scapula.
4 Pulmonary Trunk.
5 Left Main Pulmonary Artery.

Axial CTPA – pulmonary phase.

7.11
1 Right Superior Orbital ridge.
2 Right Ramus of Mandible.
3 Right Coranoid Process of Mandible.
4 Right Mastiod Air Cells.
5 Crista Galli.

Occipitofrontal skull radiograph.

The mandible has several named parts: the body which supports the teeth, the angle which marks the transition to the more vertical ramus (where masseter attaches). Superiorly the coranoid process is seen anteriorly and the condyle (or head of mandible) posteriorly.

7.12
1   Left SacroIliac Joint.
2   Right 11th Rib.
3   Left Transverse Process of L2.
4   Right Pedicle of L4.
5   Left Inferior Articular Process (Facet) of L3.

AP lumbar spine radiograph.

The spinal canal is enclosed by the neural arch of the vertebrae. The neural arch between spinous process and transverse process is the lamina, between transverse process and body is the pedicle.

7.13
1   Right Sartorius Muscle.
2   Right Femoral Artery.
3   Rectum.
4   Left Greater Trochanter.
5   Left Obturator Internus Muscle.

Axial contrast enhanced CT hip.

The vessels can be differentiated from the muscles due to the contrast within. From lateral to medial the order is femoral nerve, artery, vein. The femoral vein is closely associated to the deep inguinal lymph nodes and is therefore a useful marker when looking for lymphadenopathy.

7.14
1   **Left Main Bronchu**s.
2   Right 1st Rib.
3   Left Costophrenic Angle.
4   Right 5th Rib (Posterior).
5   Aortic Knuckle.

PA chest radiograph.

7.15
1   Left Lateral Mass of C1 (Atlas).
2   Neural Arch of C1 (Atlas).
3   Left Upper Incisor.
4   Odontoid Process of C2 (Dens).
5   Right Ramus of Mandible.

Odontoid peg radiograph (open mouth projection).

Fractures of the odontoid process are classified according to the level of injury.

Type I occur at the tip and are often stable.

Type II are through the junction of the peg and the body.

Type III extend into the body of the Axis (C2). Type II and III fractures are unstable and require stabilisation and assessment with CT imaging.

7.16
1 Left Calcaneum.
2 Base of Left 5th Metatarsal.
3 Left Cuboid.
4 Left Navicular.
5 Os Trigonum of Left Ankle.

Lateral radiograph left ankle.

Os Trigonum is an accessory bone found just posterior to the talus. It is present in between 2.5 and 14% of normal feet.

7.17
1 Manubriosternal Junction (Sternal Angle, Angle of Louis).
2 Cerebellum.
3 Mandible.
4 Fat in Marrow of Clivus.
5 Ligamentum Flavum (Yellow Ligaments).

Sagittal T2W MRI.

The ligamenta flava are so called for their distinctive appearance. They connect the lamina of vertebrae from the axis all the way to the sacrum.

7.18
1 Bladder.
2 Portal Vein.
3 **Right Internal Oblique Muscle**.
4 **Ascending Colon**.
5 Right Common Iliac Vein.

Coronal T2W MRI abdomen.

The portal vein is the continuation of the superior mesenteric vein (SMV). It becomes the portal vein at the confluence of the SMV and the splenic vein behind the neck of the pancreas. This is an important landmark during USS of the abdomen. The portal vein divides into left and right branches at the porta hepatis.

7.19
1 Clivus.
2 Right Zygomatic Arch.
3 Left Foramen Ovale.
4 Right Foramen Spinosum.
5 Right Lambdoid Suture.

Axial CT maxillary sinuses bone windows.

The foramen ovale lies within the greater wing of the sphenoid and transmits the mandibular nerve, lesser petrosal nerve, accessory meningeal artery and an emissary vein. The foramen spinosum also lies in the greater wing of the sphenoid and transmits the middle meningeal vessels.

7.20

1 **Azygos Vein.**
2 **Right Erector Spinae Muscle.**
3 Left Axillary Vein.
4 Spine of Right Scapula.
5 Right Pectoralis Major Muscle.

Axial contrast enhanced CT upper chest.

The subclavian vessels become the axillary vessels when they cross the outer border of the 1st rib. Contrast can be seen in the right axillary/subclavian vein which is causing an artefact effect.

Exam 8

8.1

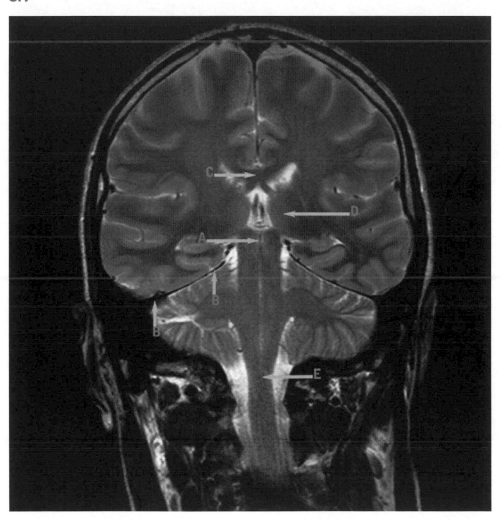

Answer the following questions.

1 Name structure 'A'.
2 Name structure 'B'.
3 Name structure 'C'.
4 Name structure 'D'.
5 Name structure 'E'.

8.2

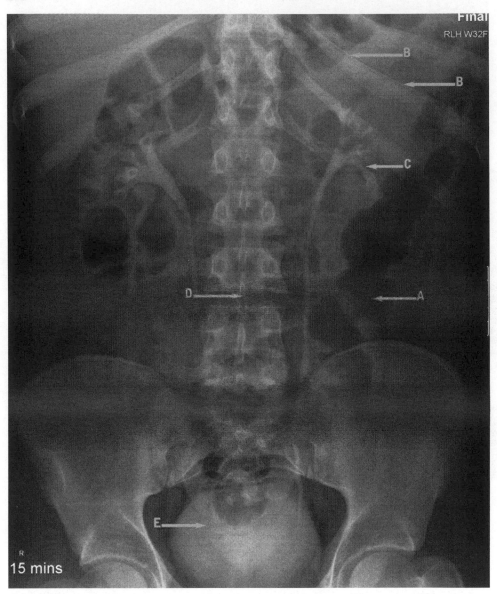

Answer the following questions.

1 Where is the gas seen at 'A'?
2 Name structure 'B'.
3 Name structure 'C'.
4 Name structure 'D'.
5 Name structure 'E'.

8.3

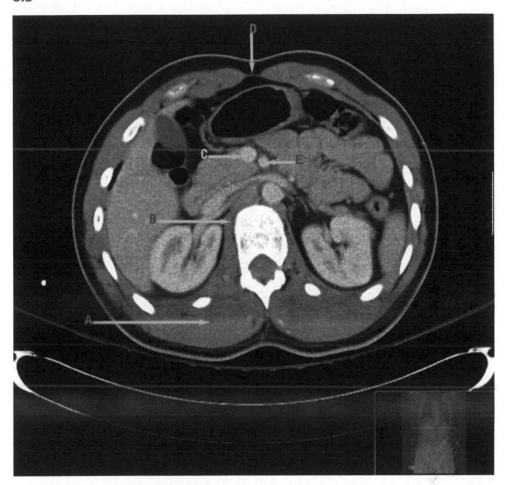

Answer the following questions.

1   Name structure 'A'.
2   Name structure 'B'.
3   Name structure 'C'.
4   Name structure 'D'.
5   Name structure 'E'.

8.4

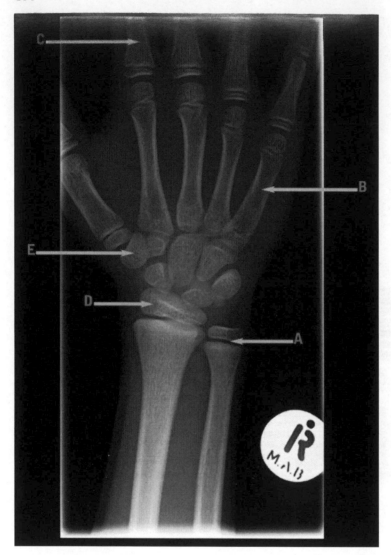

Answer the following questions.

1 Name structure 'A'.
2 Name structure 'B'.
3 Name structure 'C'.
4 Name structure 'D'.
5 Name structure 'E'.

8.5

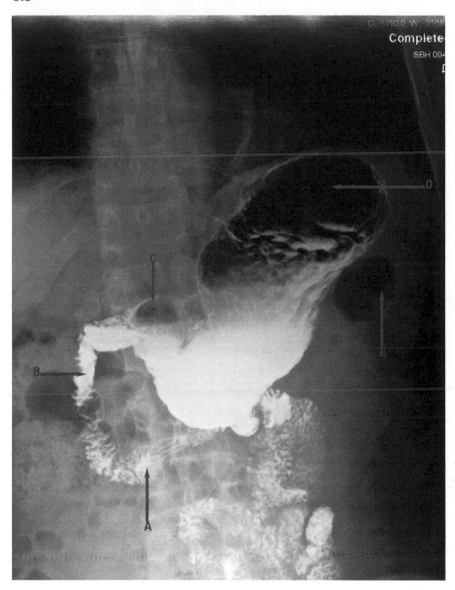

Answer the following questions.

1   Name structure 'A'.
2   Name structure 'B'.
3   Name structure 'C'.
4   Name structure 'D'.
5   Name structure 'E'.

8.6

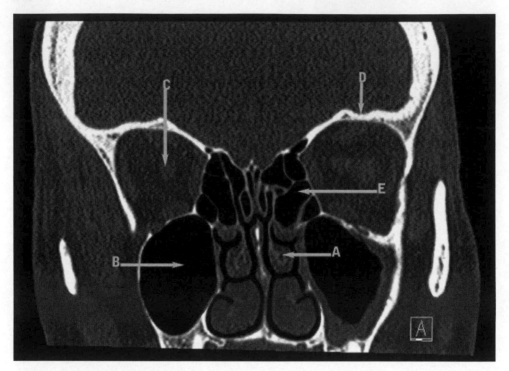

Answer the following questions.

1   **Name structure 'A'.**
2   Name structure 'B'.
3   Name structure 'C'.
4   Name structure 'D'.
5   Name structure 'E'.

8.7

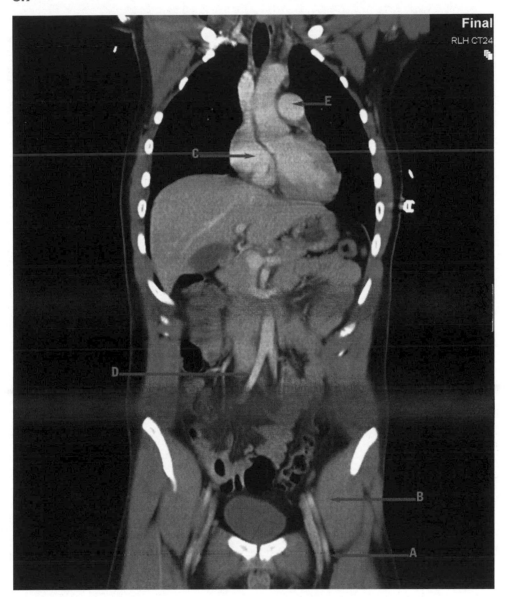

Answer the following questions.

1   Name structure 'A'.
2   Name structure 'B'.
3   Name structure 'C'.
4   Name structure 'D'.
5   Name structure 'E'.

8.8

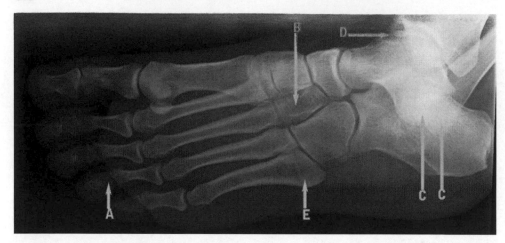

Answer the following questions.

1   Name structure 'A'.
2   Name structure 'B'.
3   Name structure 'C'.
4   Name structure 'D'.
5   Name structure 'E'.

8.9

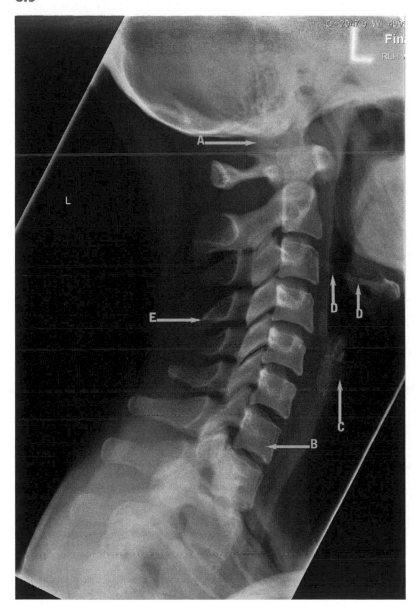

Answer the following questions.

1 Name structure 'A'.
2 Name structure 'B'.
3 Name structure 'C'.
4 Name structure 'D'.
5 Name structure 'E'.

8.10

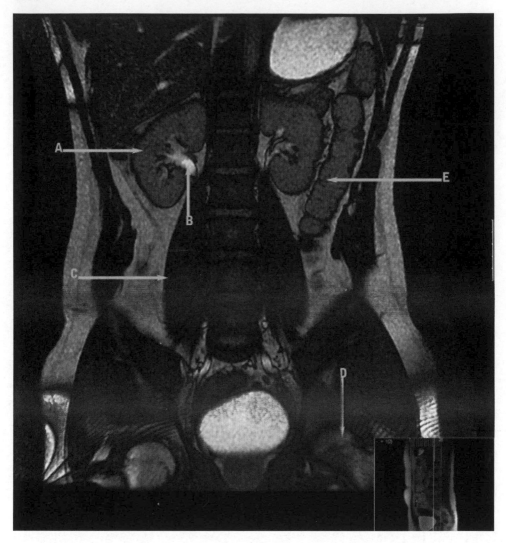

Answer the following questions.

1   Name structure 'A'.
2   Name structure 'B'.
3   Name structure 'C'.
4   Name structure 'D'.
5   Name structure 'E'.

8.11

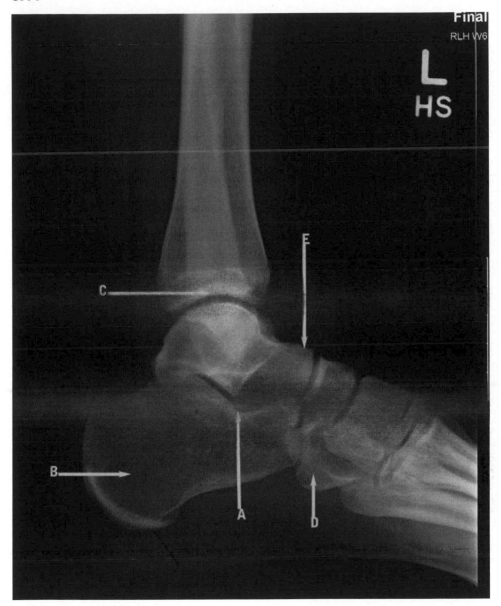

Answer the following questions.

1   Name structure 'A'.
2   Name structure 'B'.
3   Name structure 'C'.
4   Name structure 'D'.
5   Name structure 'E'.

8.12

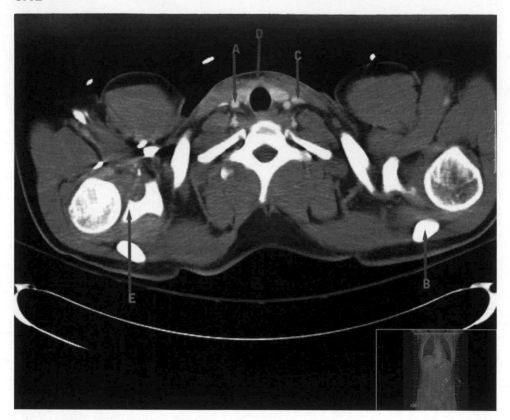

Answer the following questions.

1   Name structure 'A'.
2   Name structure 'B'.
3   Name structure 'C'.
4   Name structure 'D'.
5   Name structure 'E'.

8.13

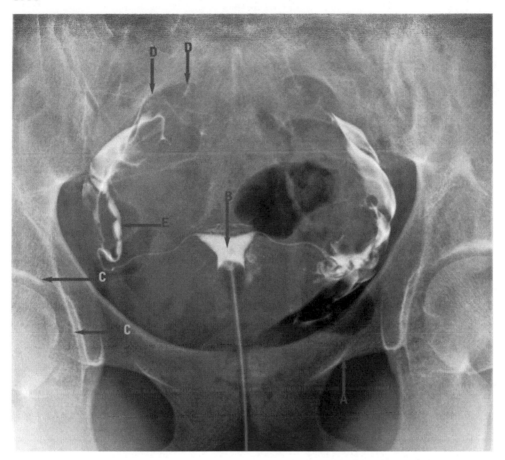

Answer the following questions.

1   Name structure 'A'.
2   Name structure 'B'.
3   Name structure 'C'.
4   Name structure 'D'.
5   Name structure 'E'.

8.14

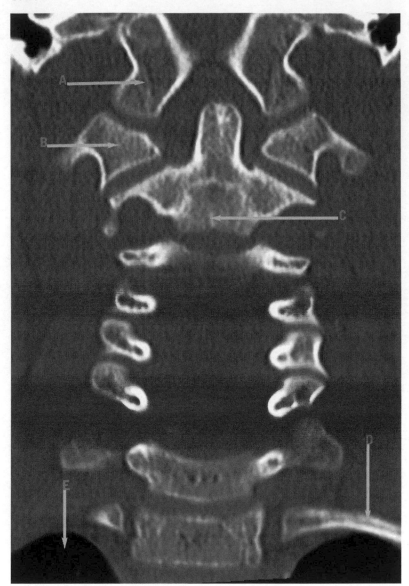

Answer the following questions.

1 Name structure 'A'.
2 Name structure 'B'.
3 Name structure 'C'.
4 Name structure 'D'.
5 Name structure 'E'.

8.15

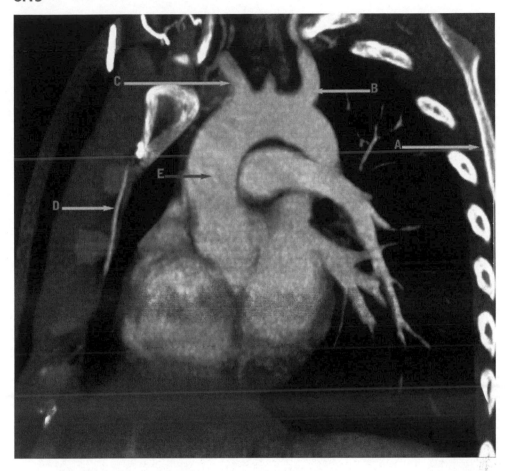

Answer the following questions.

1   Name structure 'A'.
2   Name structure 'B'.
3   Name structure 'C'.
4   Name structure 'D'.
5   Name structure 'E'.

8.16

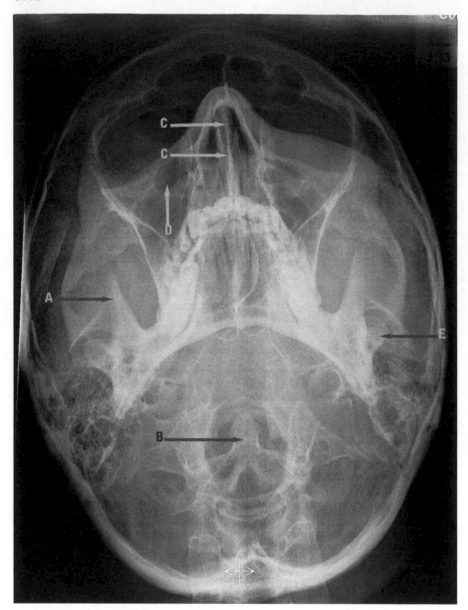

Answer the following questions.

1 Name structure 'A'.
2 Name structure 'B'.
3 Name structure 'C'.
4 Name structure 'D'.
5 Name structure 'E'.

8.17

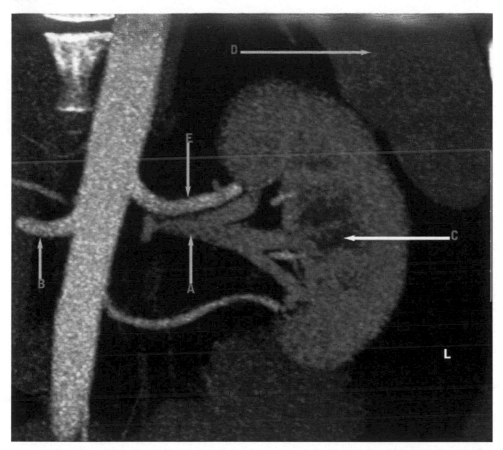

Answer the following questions.

1 Name structure 'A'.
2 Name structure 'B'.
3 Name structure 'C'.
4 Name structure 'D'.
5 Name structure 'E'.

8.18

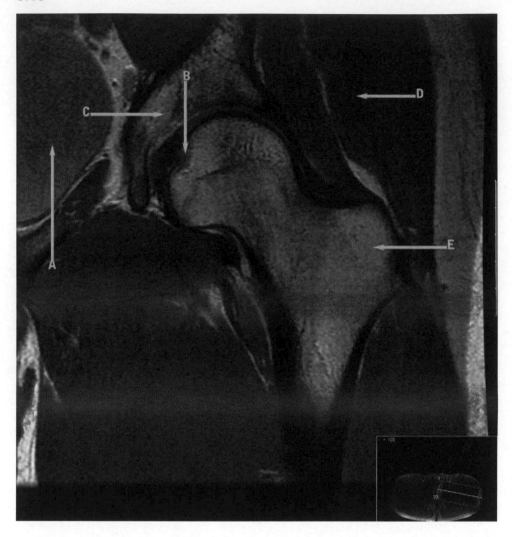

Answer the following questions.

1   Name structure 'A'.
2   Name structure 'B'.
3   Name structure 'C'.
4   Name structure 'D'.
5   Name structure 'E'.

8.19

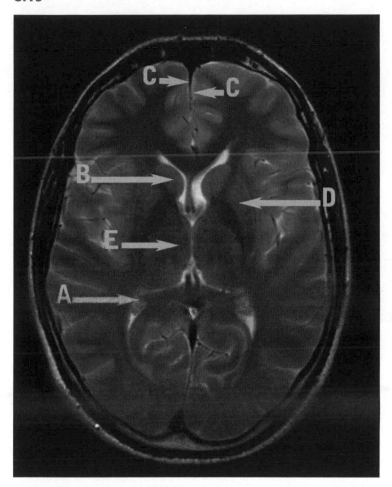

Answer the following questions.

1   Name structure 'A'.
2   Name structure 'B'.
3   Name structure 'C'.
4   Name structure 'D'.
5   Name structure 'E'.

8.20

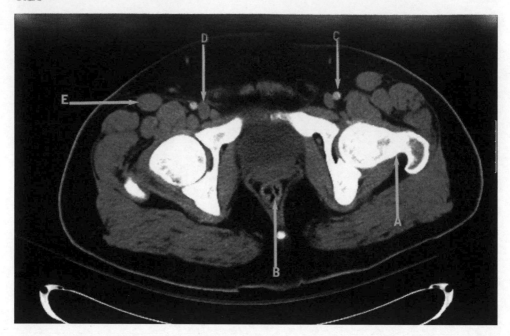

Answer the following questions.

1   Name structure 'A'.
2   Name structure 'B'.
3   Name structure 'C'.
4   Name structure 'D'.
5   Name structure 'E'.

Answers

8.1
1 Aqueduct of Sylvius.
2 Tentorium Cerebelli.
3 Corpus Callosum.
4 Thalamus.
5 Spinal Cord.

Sagittal T2W MRI.

The aqueduct of Sylvius connects the 3rd ventricle to the 4th ventricle. The 4th ventricle can be seen in this image in its distinctive diamond shape in cross section. The caudal tip of the 4th ventricle, or obex, represents the imaginary dividing line between the medulla and the spinal cord and lies at the level of the foramen magnum.

8.2
1 Descending Colon.
2 Left 10th Rib.
3 Left Inferior Pole Minor Calyx.
4 Spinous Process of L3.
5 Bladder.

IVU excretory phase.

The large bowel can be distinguished from small bowel on x-ray due to the wall features and position. A distinctive haustral pattern is seen in large bowel; the haustra do not fully cross the bowel. The valvulae conniventes of the small bowel traverse the whole distance. The maximum normal diameter for large bowel is 55mm, the small bowel 35mm.

8.3
1 Right Erector Spinae Muscle.
2 Right Crus of Diaphragm.
3 Superior Mesenteric Vein.
4 Linea Alba.
5 Superior Mesenteric Artery.

Axial contrast enhanced CT abdomen.

The linea alba is formed by the aponeurosis of the abdominal wall muscles. It separates the rectus abdominis muscles and is composed of fibrous tissue only, containing no nerves or vessels. The erector spinae is a muscle group formed from three muscles (lateral to medial): iliocostalis, longissimus and spinalis. These can be remembered by the mnemonic 'I Long for Spinach'.

8.4

1   Metaphysis of Right Distal Ulna (Or Epiphyseal Plate).
2   Diaphysis of Right Little Finger Metacarpal.
3   Diaphysis of Right index Finger Proximal Phalanx.
4   Epiphysis of Right Distal Radius.
5   Right Trapezium.

AP wrist radiograph.

This child is approximately aged 12.

8.5

1   3rd (Horizontal) Part of Duodenum.
2   2nd (Descending) Part of Duodenum.
3   Duodenal Cap (1st Part of Duodenum).
4   Fundus of Stomach.
5   Gas at Splenic Flexure.

Double contrast barium meal.

The duodenum is divided into 4 parts. All but the 1st are retroperitoneal, the 4th part enters the peritoneal cavity at the duodenojejunal Flexure (DJ flexure), surrounded by a peritoneal fold called the ligament of Treitz to become the jejunum.

8.6

1   Left Middle Nasal Concha (Turbinate).
2   Right Maxillary Sinus.
3   **Right Optic Nerve**.
4   **Left Supraorbital Margin (Frontal Bone)**.
5   Left Ethmoidal Air Cells.

Coronal CT Orbits.

8.7

1   Left Common Femoral Artery.
2   Left Iliopsoas Muscle.
3   Right Atrium.
4   Right Common Iliac Artery.
5   Pulmonary Trunk.

Coronal CT pelvis.

8.8

1   4th Middle Phalanx.
2   Lateral Cuneiform.
3   Lateral Malleolus of Fibula.
4   Talus.
5   Base of 5th metatarsal.

Oblique radiograph of foot.

8.9
1   Occipital Condyle.
2   Body of C7 vertebra.
3   Cricoid Cartilage.
4   Greater Horn of Hyoid Bone.
5   Spinous Process of C4 Vertebra.

Lateral radiograph cervical spine.

The cricoid cartilage forms the only complete cartilaginous ring of the trachea. It lies inferiorly to the thyroid cartilage to which it is attached by the cricothyroid ligament in the midline and posteriorly by the two cricothyroid joints.

8.10
1   Medulla of Right Kidney.
2   Right Renal Pelvis.
3   Right Psoas Muscle.
4   Head of Left Femur.
5   Descending colon.

T2W coronal MRI abdomen/pelvis.

Whilst the caecum, transverse and sigmoid colon are intraperitoneal structures, the ascending and descending parts of the colon are retroperitoneal. It is closely related to the lateral border of the left kidney.

8.11
1   **Left Sinus Tarsi.**
2   **Left Calcaneum.**
3   Articular Surface of Left Tibia.
4   Left Cuboid.
5   Head of Left Talus.

Lateral ankle/foot radiograph.

The sinus tarsi is a depression on the lateral side of the tarsus and is at the same level as the lateral malleolus. It is a canal through the talocalcaneal joint through which runs the interosseus talocalcaneal ligament.

8.12
1   Right Common Carotid Artery.
2   Left Scapular Spine.
3   Left Internal Jugular Vein.
4   Isthmus of Thyroid.
5   Right Glenoid.

Axial contrast enhanced CT neck.

8.13
1   **Left Superior Pubic Ramus.**
2   **Body of Uterus.**
3   Right Acetabulum.
4   Sacral Foramen.
5   Ampulla of Right Uterine (Fallopian) Tube.

Hysterosalpingogram (HSG).

An HSG is used to assess the patency of the uterine tubes as well as to outline any uterine structural abnormalities.

8.14
1   Right Occipital Condyle.
2   Right Lateral Mass of C1.
3   Body of C2.
4   Left 1st Rib.
5   Apex of Right Lung.

Coronal CT cervical spine.

The C1 vertebra, or atlas, is named after the mythical giant who supported the globe on his shoulders, as it supports the globe of the head. Whilst it has no body, it has two lateral masses which articulate with the occipital condyles above and the C2 vertebra (axis) below.

8.15
1   Blade of Scapula.
2   Left Subclavian Artery.
3   Brachiocephalic Trunk.
4   Internal Thoracic Artery.
5   Ascending Aorta.

Sagittal CTA chest.

8.16
1   Right Coronoid Process of Mandible.
2   Odontoid Process of C2.
3   Nasal Septum.
4   Right Infraorbital Foramen.
5   Left Condyle of Mandible.

Occipitomental radiograph facial bones.

The infraorbital foramen transmits the infraorbital vein, nerve and artery. The nerve is a branch of the maxillary nerve, itself a branch of the trigeminal nerve (CNV).

8.17
1   Left Renal Vein.
2   Right Renal Artery.

3 Renal Medulla of Left Kidney.
4 **Spleen.**
5 **Left Renal Artery.**

CTA left kidney.

Note the small side marker on the image.

8.18
1 Bladder.
2 Fovea of Left Femoral Head.
3 Left Acetabulum.
4 Left Gluteus Medius.
5 Left Greater Trochanter.

Coronal MRI hip.

The fovea is a depression in the cartilage of the head which is the point of attachment of the ligamentum teres. The gluteus medius muscle can be seen attaching to the greater trochanter. It lies lateral to the gluteus minimus which is also clearly seen on this image. Other muscles which attach at the greater trochanter include gluteus minimus, piriformis, the gemelli muscles and obturator externus and internus. The gluteus maximus attaches below the trochanter at the iliotibial tract.

8.19
1 Right Choroid Plexus.
2 Head of Right Caudate Nucleus.
3 Falx Cerebri.
4 Putamen.
5 Thalamus.

Axial T2W MRI brain.

8.20
1 Left Femoral Neck.
2 Rectum.
3 Left Femoral Artery.
4 Right Femoral Vein.
5 Right Sartorius Muscle.

Axial contrast enhanced CT lower limbs.

Exam 9

9.1

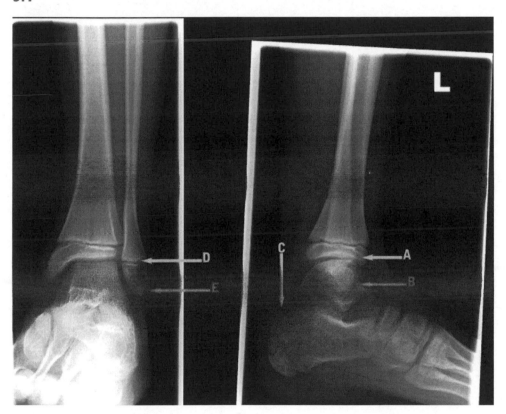

Answer the following questions.

1   Name structure 'A'.
2   Name structure 'B'.
3   What attaches at 'C'?
4   Name structure 'D'.
5   Name structure 'E'.

9.2

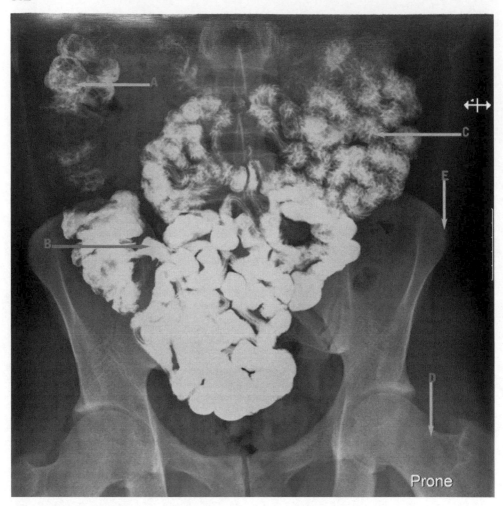

Answer the following questions.

1   Name structure 'A'.
2   Name structure 'B'.
3   Name structure 'C'.
4   Name structure 'D'.
5   Name structure 'E'.

9.3

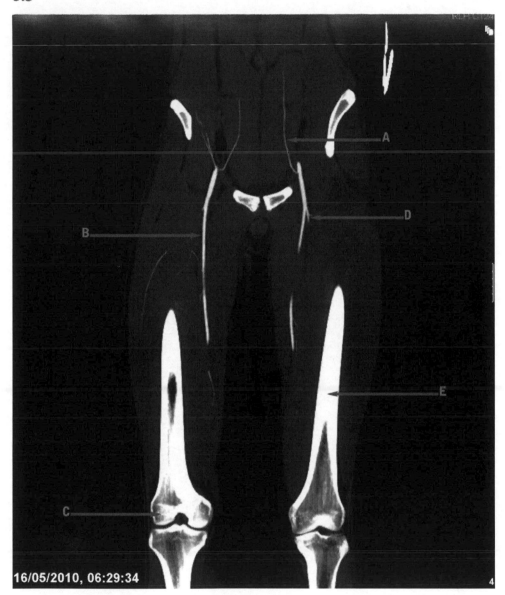

Answer the following questions.

1 Name structure 'A'.
2 Name structure 'B'.
3 Name structure 'C'.
4 Name structure 'D'.
5 Name structure 'E'.

9.4

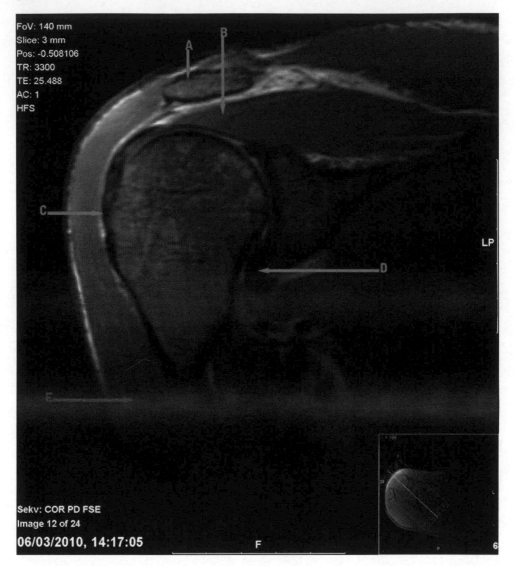

FoV: 140 mm
Slice: 3 mm
Pos: -0.508106
TR: 3300
TE: 25.488
AC: 1
HFS

Sekv: COR PD FSE
Image 12 of 24
06/03/2010, 14:17:05

Answer the following questions.

1   Name structure 'A'.
2   Name structure 'B'.
3   Name structure 'C'.
4   Name structure 'D'.
5   Name structure 'E'.

9.5

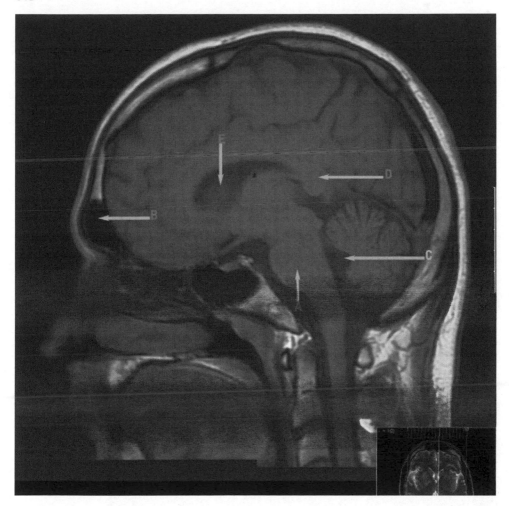

Answer the following questions.

1   Name structure 'A'.
2   Name structure 'B'.
3   Name structure 'C'.
4   Name structure 'D'.
5   Name structure 'E'.

9.6

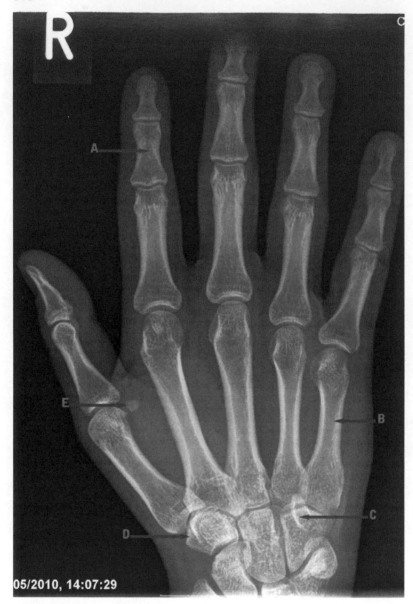

Answer the following questions.

1 Name structure 'A'.
2 Name structure 'B'.
3 Name structure 'C'.
4 Name structure 'D'.
5 Name structure 'E'.

9.7

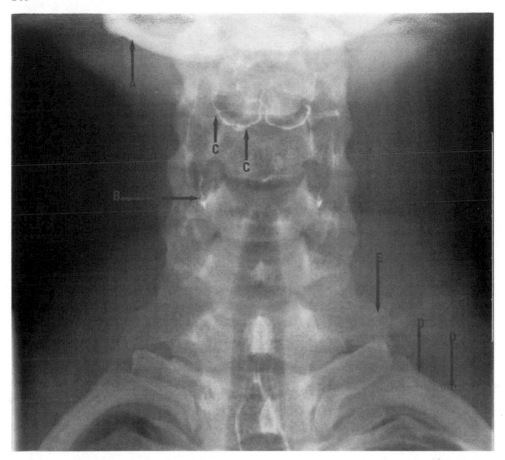

Answer the following questions.

1 Name structure 'A'.
2 Name structure 'B'.
3 Name structure 'C'.
4 Name structure 'D'.
5 Name structure 'E'.

9.8

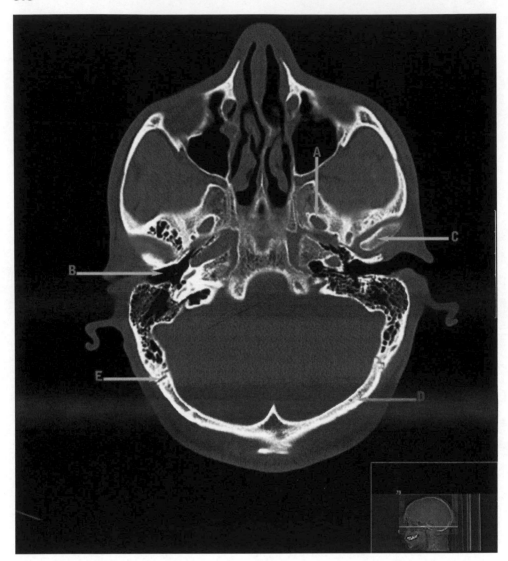

Answer the following questions.

1 Name structure 'A'.
2 Name structure 'B'.
3 Name structure 'C'.
4 Name structure 'D'.
5 Name structure 'E'.

9.9

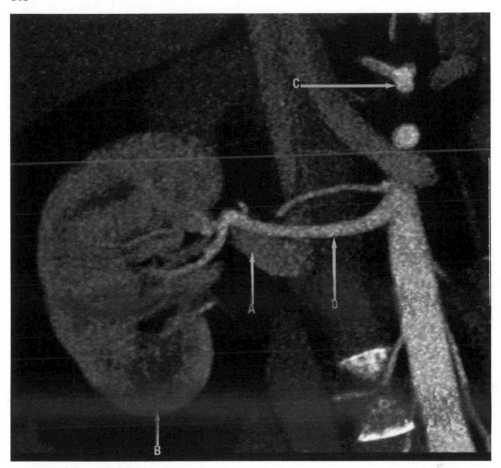

Answer the following questions.

1 Name structure 'A'.
2 Name structure 'B'.
3 Name structure 'C'.
4 Name structure 'D'.
5 At what level does 'D' normally arise?

9.10

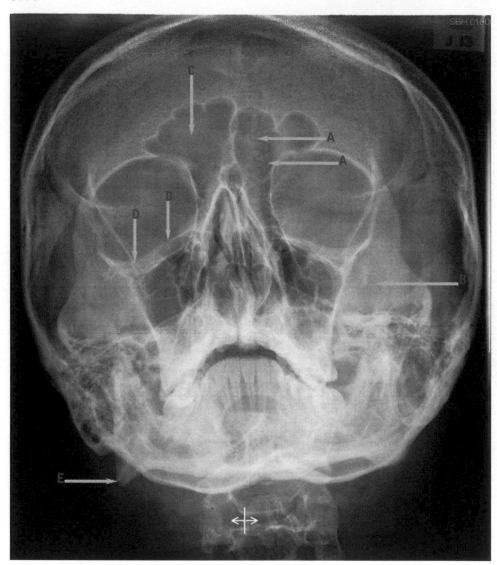

Answer the following questions.

1   Name structure 'A'.
2   Name structure 'B'.
3   Name structure 'C'.
4   Name structure 'D'.
5   Name structure 'E'.

9.11

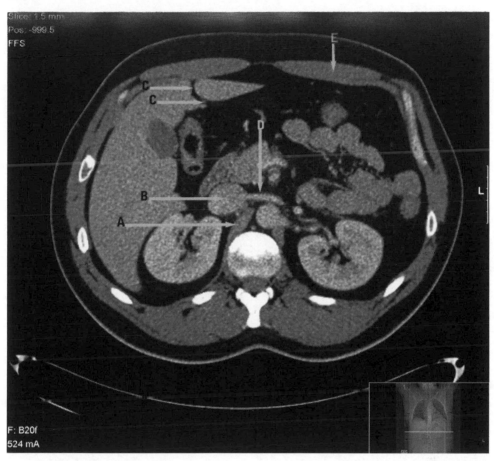

Answer the following questions.

1   Name structure 'A'.
2   Name structure 'B'.
3   Name structure 'C'.
4   Name structure 'D'.
5   Name structure 'E'.

9.12

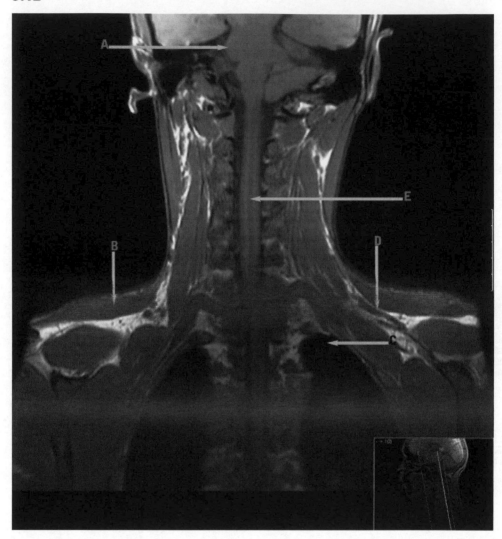

Answer the following questions.

1   Name structure 'A'.
2   Name structure 'B'.
3   Name structure 'C'.
4   Name structure 'D'.
5   Name structure 'E'.

9.13

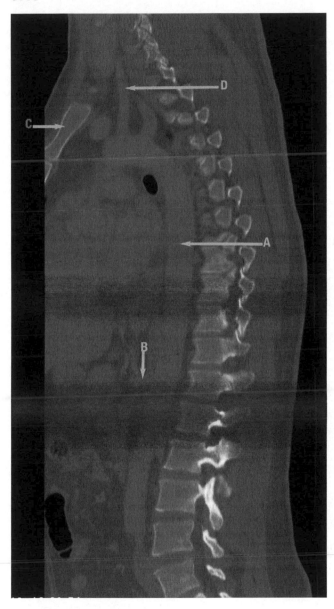

Answer the following questions.

1   Name structure 'A'.
2   Name structure 'B'.
3   Name structure 'C'.
4   Name structure 'D'.
5   At what level does 'B' usually arise?

9.14

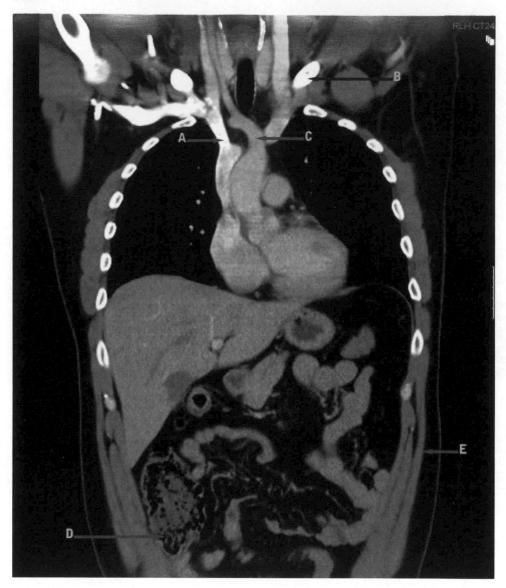

Answer the following questions.

1 Name structure 'A'.
2 Name structure 'B'.
3 Name structure 'C'.
4 Name structure 'D'.
5 Name structure 'E'.

9.15

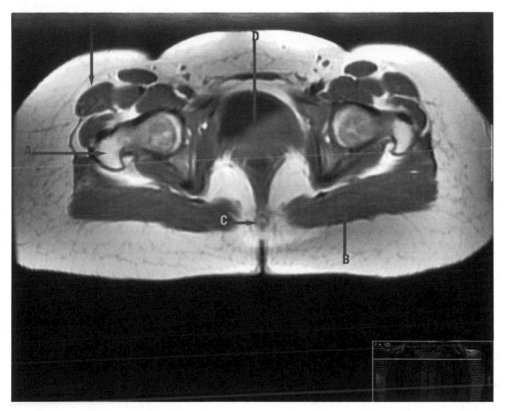

Answer the following questions.

1 Name structure 'A'.
2 Name structure 'B'.
3 Name structure 'C'.
4 Name structure 'D'.
5 Name structure 'E'.

9.16

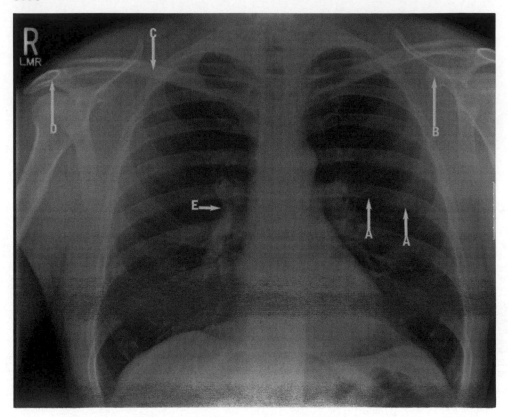

Answer the following questions.

1 Name structure 'A'.
2 Name structure 'B'.
3 Name structure 'C'.
4 Name structure 'D'.
5 Name structure 'E'.

9.17

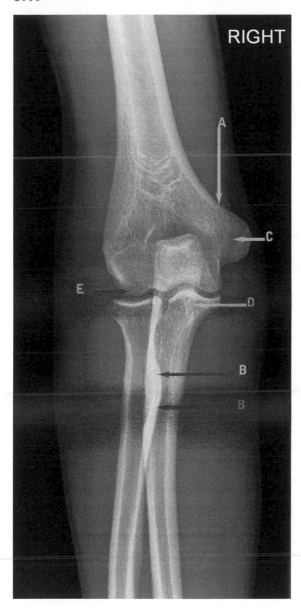

RIGHT

Answer the following questions.

1 Name structure 'A'.
2 Name structure 'B'.
3 Name structure 'C'.
4 Name structure 'D'.
5 Name structure 'E'.

9.18

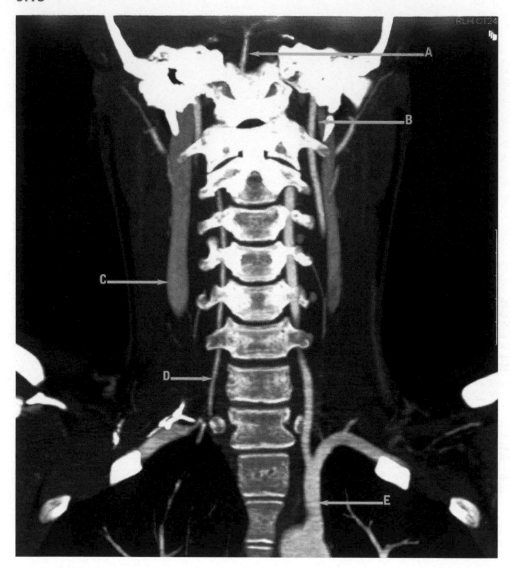

Answer the following questions.

1 Name structure 'A'.
2 Name structure 'B'.
3 Name structure 'C'.
4 Name structure 'D'.
5 Name structure 'E'.

9.19

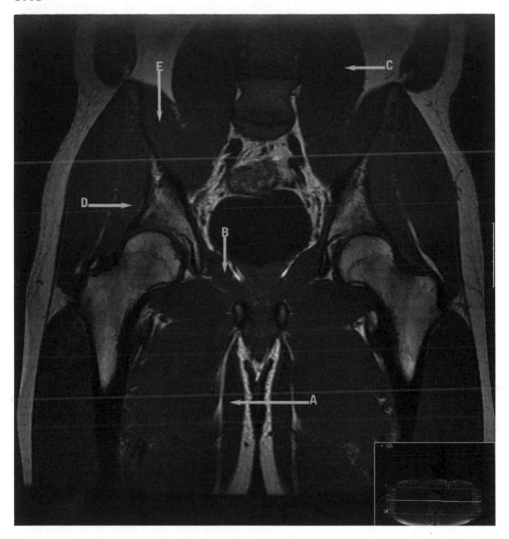

Answer the following questions.

1 Name structure 'A'.
2 Name structure 'B'.
3 Name structure 'C'.
4 Name structure 'D'.
5 Name structure 'E'.

9.20

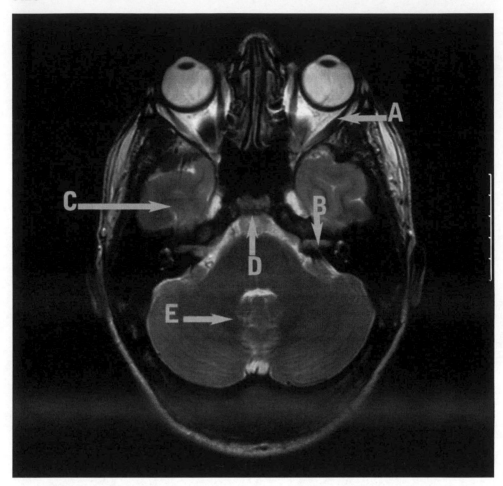

Answer the following questions.

1   Name structure 'A'.
2   Name structure 'B'.
3   Name structure 'C'.
4   Name structure 'D'.
5   Name structure 'E'.

Answers

9.1
1 Left Distal Tibial Epiphysis.
2 Left Talus.
3 Left Achilles Tendon (Tendo Calcaneus).
4 Left Distal Fibula Epiphyseal Line (Growth Plate).
5 Left Lateral Malleolus.

AP and lateral radiograph paediatric ankle.

The Achilles tendon arises from the aponeuroses of the gastrocnemius and soleus muscles.

Achilles was held by the heel as he was dipped in the river Styx by his mother, hence his vulnerability at that point.

9.2
1 Ascending Colon.
2 Terminal Ileum.
3 Jejunum.
4 Left Femoral Neck.
5 Left Anterior superior Iliac Spine (ASIS).

Barium follow through.

The anterior superior iliac spine (ASIS) represents the most anterior part of the iliac crest. It is the lateral site of insertion of the inguinal ligament and as such is an important landmark. It is also a site of insertion of the sartorius muscle and the tensor fasciae latae.

9.3
1 Left Inferior Epigastric Artery.
2 Right Superficial Femoral Artery.
3 Right Lateral Epicondyle of Femur.
4 Left Profunda Femoris Artery.
5 Shaft of Right Femur.

Coronal CTA lower limbs.

The bifurcation of the common femoral artery can be seen. The profunda femoris supplies all of the thigh muscles. Its branches are the medial and lateral circumflex arteries and four perforating arteries which supply the adductors and hamstrings. The inferior epigastric artery arises from the external iliac artery at the inguinal ligament.

9.4

1   **Right Acromion.**
2   **Right Supraspinatus Muscle.**
3   Right Greater Tuberosity of Humerus.
4   Right Glenoid Labrum.
5   Right Deltoid Muscle.

Coronal MRI right shoulder.

The shoulder joint is reliant on its muscles for stability. The relatively shallow glenoid is deepened slightly by the labrum surrounding it, but the main stabilisers of the joint are the rotator cuff muscles: supraspinatus, infraspinatus, teres minor and subscapularis. These may be remembered by the mnemonic SITS.

9.5

1   Pons.
2   Frontal Sinus.
3   4th Ventricle.
4   Splenium of Corpus Callosum.
5   Lateral Ventricle.

Sagittal T1W MRI brain.

9.6

1   Middle Phalanx of Right Index Finger.
2   Right 5th Metacarpal.
3   Hook of Right Hamate.
4   Right Trapezium.
5   Sesamoid Bone of Right Hand.

Dorsopalmar radiograph right hand.

Sesamoid bones are found where tendons pass over a joint. In the hand there are commonly two found at the 1st metacarpophalangeal joint. They lie within the tendons of adductor pollicis and abductor pollicis brevis. The pisiform bone of the wrist is a sesamoid as is the patella.

9.7

1   Mandible.
2   Right Piriform Fossa.
3   Right Vallecula.
4   Left 1st Rib.
5   Left Transverse Process of C7.

Double contrast AP radiograph of pharynx (vallecula view).

A common view taken during barium swallow studies, the double contrast is achieved by asking the patient to 'puff out the cheeks', forcing air into the pharynx against a closed epiglottis.

9.8
1   Left Foramen Ovale.
2   Right External Acoustic Canal.
3   Left Condyle of Mandible.
4   Occipital Bone.
5   Lambdoid Suture (Right Aspect).

Axial CT base of skull bone windows.

The lambdoid suture lies between the squamous part of the occipital and the parietal bones. It meets the sagittal suture in the midline at a point called the lambda. The coronal suture lies anteriorly between the frontal and parietal bones, it meets at a midline point called the bregma from which the sagittal suture passes posteriorly.

9.9
1   Right Renal Vein.
2   Inferior Pole Renal Cortex Right Kidney.
3   Coeliac Axis.
4   Right Renal Artery.
5   L1.

Coronal CTA right kidney.

9.10
1   Sagittal Suture.
2   Left Zygomatic Bone.
3   Frontal Sinus.
4   Right Inferior Orbital Ridge.
5   Right Angle of Mandible.

Occipitomental skull radiograph.

The bony orbit is formed from seven bones. It is often thought of as a pyramid, with its base at the face and apex at the optic canal. The bones are: temporal (lateral and inferior wall), maxilla (inferior, medial), lacrimal (medial), ethmoid (medial), frontal (superior), sphenoid (posterior/apical) and palatine (medial, inferior).

9.11
1   Right Crus of Diaphragm.
2   Inferior Vena Cava.
3   Falciform Ligament.
4   Left Renal Vein.
5   Left Rectus Abdominis Muscle.

Axial CT abdomen.

9.12
1   Right Middle Cerebellar Peduncle.
2   Right Trapezius Muscle.
3   Apex of Left Lung.

4 Left Brachial Plexus.
5 Spinal Cord.

Coronal T1W MRI.

9.13
1 Descending (Thoracic) Aorta.
2 Coeliac Axis.
3 Manubrium.
4 Left Common Carotid Artery.
5 T12.

Parasagittal non contrast CT aorta.

The coeliac axis is the first abdominal (subdiaphragmatic) branch of the aorta. It divides into the splenic, left gastric and common hepatic arteries. These vessels and their branches supply the upper abdominal organs corresponding to the embryonic foregut.

9.14
1 Right Brachiocephalic Vein.
2 Left Clavicle.
3 Brachiocephalic Trunk.
4 Caecum.
5 Left External Oblique Muscle.

Coronal contrast enhanced CT thorax/abdomen.

9.15
1 **Right Greater Trochanter.**
2 Left Gluteus Maximus.
3 Coccyx.
4 Bladder.
5 Right Tensor Fasciae Latae Muscle.

Axial T1W MRI through femoral neck.

9.16
1 Left 7th Rib.
2 Coracoid Process of Left Scapula.
3 Right Clavicle.
4 Right Acromion Process of Scapula.
5 Right Hilar Point.

PA chest radiograph.

9.17
1 Right Medial Supracondylar Ridge.
2 Right Radial Tuberosity.
3 Medial Epicondyle of Right Humerus.

4   Coronoid Process of Right Ulna.
5   Right Capitellum.

AP elbow radiograph.

9.18
1   Basilar Artery.
2   Left Internal Carotid Artery.
3   Right Internal Jugular Vein.
4   Right Vertebral Artery.
5   Left Subclavian Artery.

Coronal CTA Reformat.

9.19
1   Right Gracilis Muscle.
2   Right Obturator Internus Muscle.
3   Left Psoas Muscle.
4   Right Gluteus Minimus Muscle.
5   Right Iliacus Muscle.

Coronal MRI hip.

9.20
1   Left Lateral Rectus Muscle.
2   Left Facial Nerve.
3   Right Temporal Lobe.
4   **Dorsum Sellae**.
5   **Dentate Nucleu**s.

Axial T2W MRI.

Exam 10

10.1

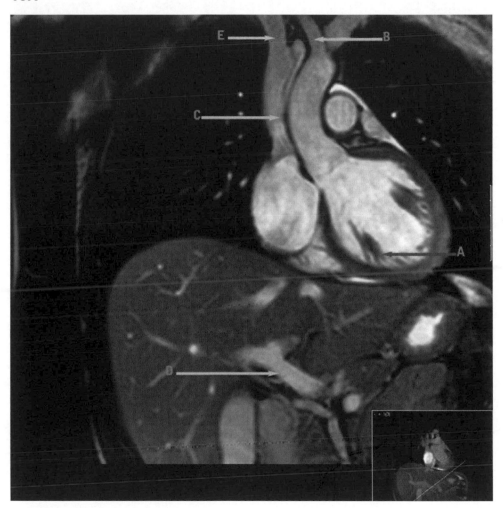

Answer the following questions.

1 Name structure 'A'.
2 Name structure 'B'.
3 Name structure 'C'.
4 Name structure 'D'.
5 Name structure 'E'.

10.2

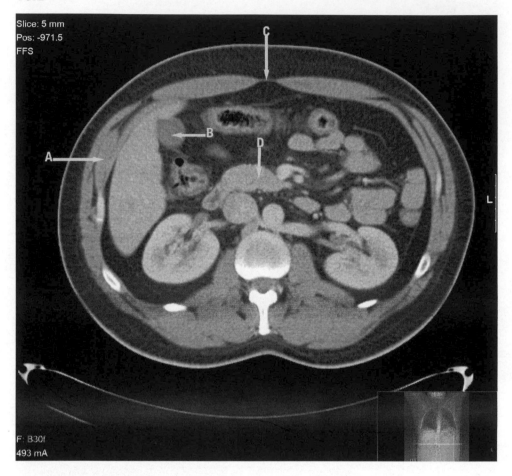

Answer the following questions.

1   Name structure 'A'.
2   Name structure 'B'.
3   Name structure 'C'.
4   Name structure 'D'.
5   What normal variant is shown?

10.3

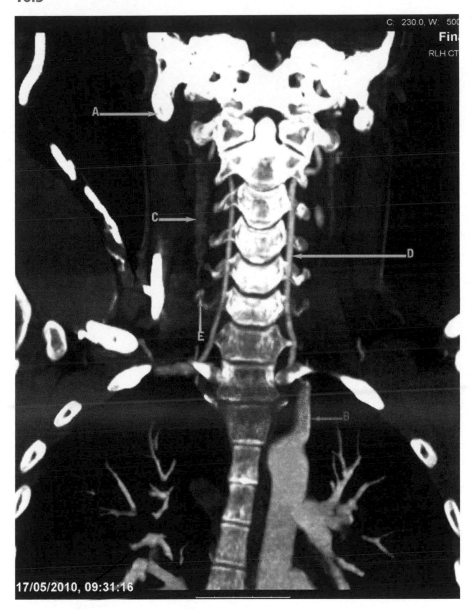

Answer the following questions.

1   Name structure 'A'.
2   Name structure 'B'.
3   Name structure 'C'.
4   Name structure 'D'.
5   Name structure 'E'.

10.4

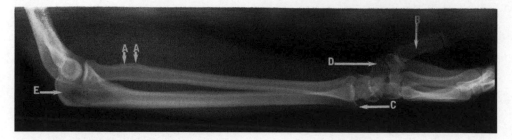

Answer the following questions.

1 Name structure 'A'.
2 Name structure 'B'.
3 Name structure 'C'.
4 Name structure 'D'.
5 Name structure 'E'.

10.5

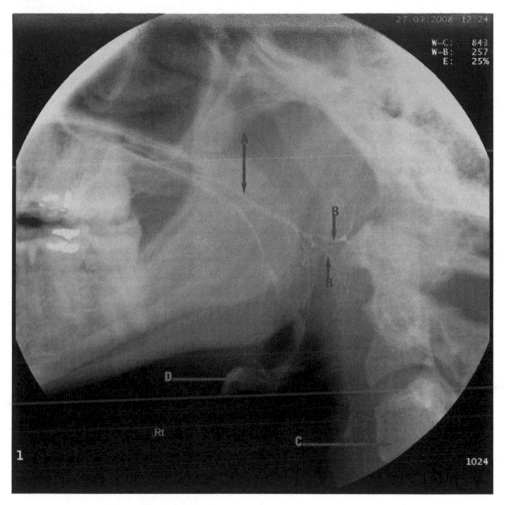

Answer the following questions.

1 Name structure 'A'.
2 Name structure 'B'.
3 Name structure 'C'.
4 Name structure 'D'.
5 Where does 'A' open?

10.6

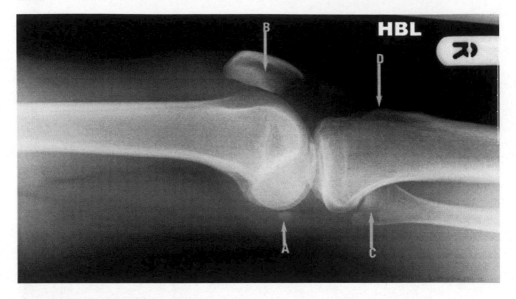

Answer the following questions.

1   Name structure 'A'.
2   Name structure 'B'.
3   Name structure 'C'.
4   Name structure 'D'.
5   **What attaches** at 'D'?

10.7

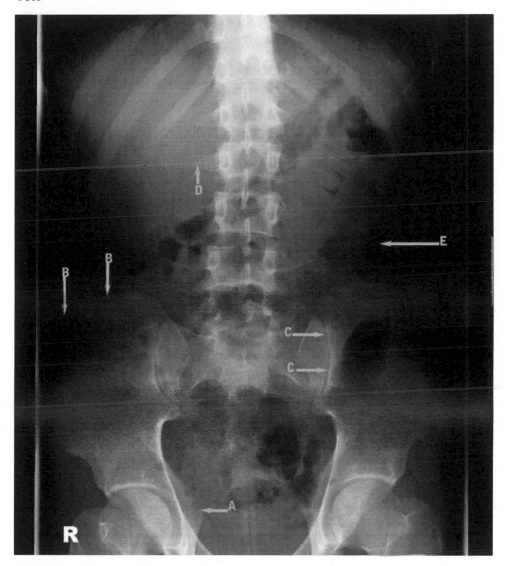

Answer the following questions.

1   Name structure 'A'.
2   Name structure 'B'.
3   Name structure 'C'.
4   Name structure 'D'.
5   Name structure 'E'.

10.8

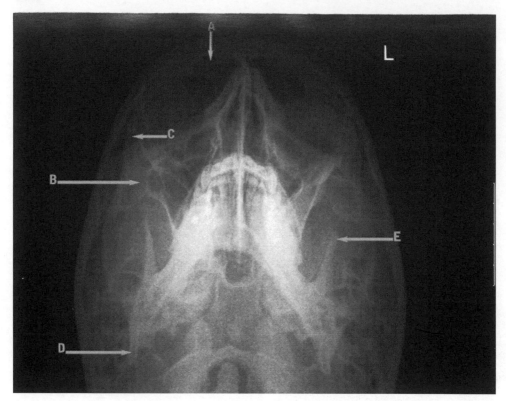

Answer the following questions.

1   Name structure 'A'.
2   Name structure 'B'.
3   Name structure 'C'.
4   Name structure 'D'.
5   Name structure 'E'.

10.9

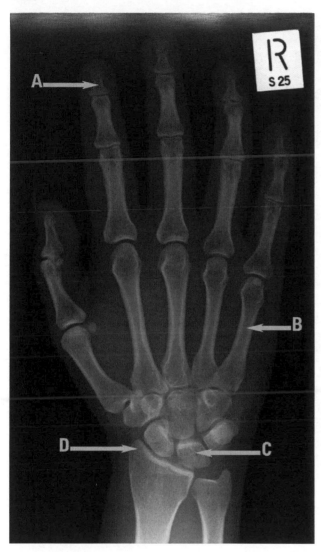

Answer the following questions.

1   Name structure 'A'.
2   Name structure 'B'.
3   Name structure 'C'.
4   Name structure 'D'.
5   Name the bony attachments of the flexor retinaculum.

10.10

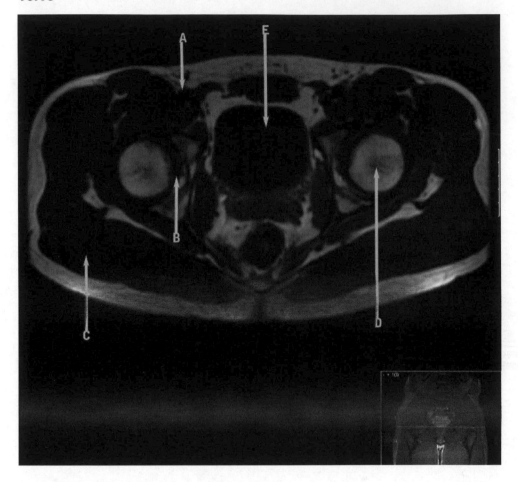

Answer the following questions.

1   Name structure 'A'.
2   Name structure 'B'.
3   Name structure 'C'.
4   Name structure 'D'.
5   Name structure 'E'.

10.11

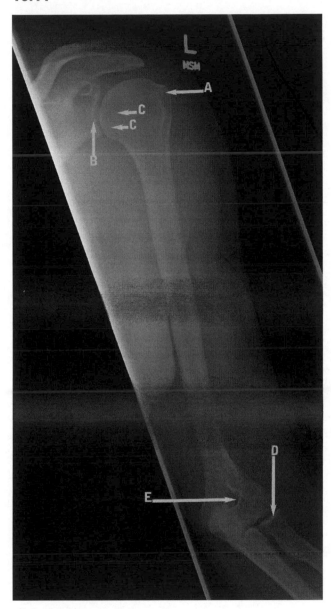

Answer the following questions.

1   Name structure 'A'.
2   Name structure 'B'.
3   Name structure 'C'.
4   Name structure 'D'.
5   Name structure 'E'.

10.12

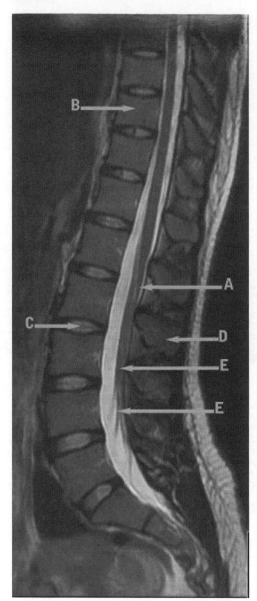

Answer the following questions.

1   Name structure 'A'.
2   Name structure 'B'.
3   Name structure 'C'.
4   Name structure 'D'.
5   Name structure 'E'.

10.13

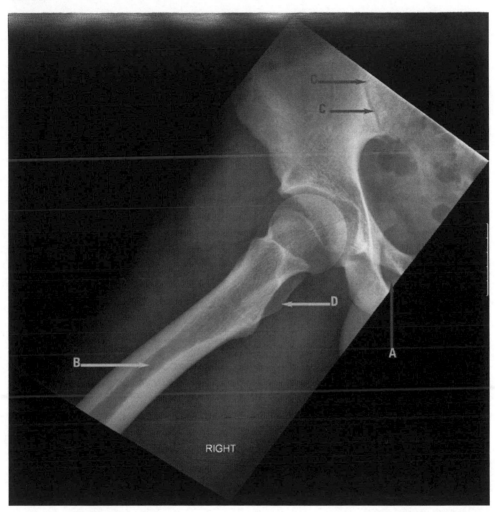

Answer the following questions.

1   Name structure 'A'.
2   Name structure 'B'.
3   Name structure 'C'.
4   Name structure 'D'.
5   What attaches at 'D'?

10.14

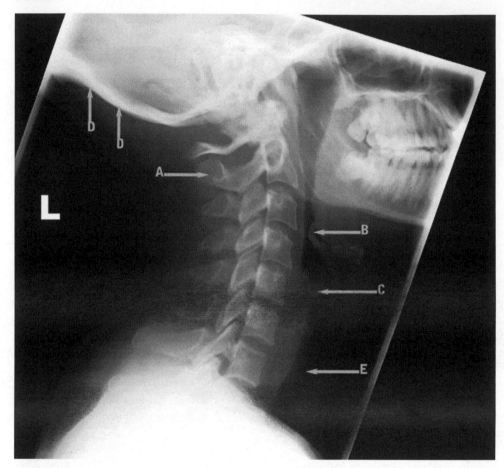

Answer the following questions.

1   Name structure 'A'.
2   Name structure 'B'.
3   Name structure 'C'.
4   Name structure 'D'.
5   Name structure 'E'.

10.15

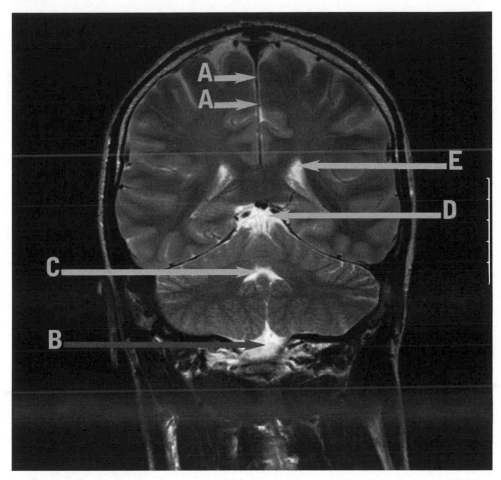

Answer the following questions.

1 Name structure 'A'.
2 Name structure 'B'.
3 Name structure 'C'.
4 Name structure 'D'.
5 Name structure 'E'.

10.16

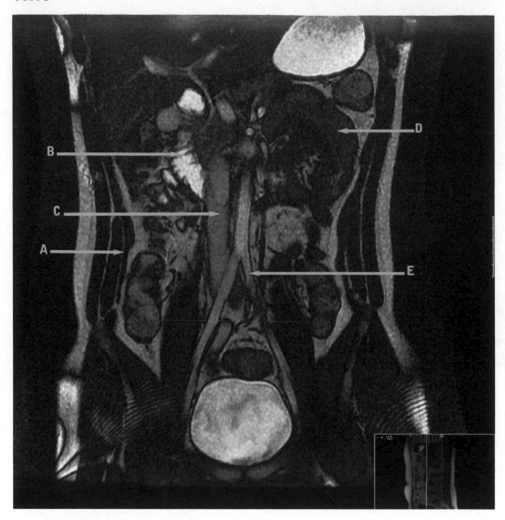

Answer the following questions.

1   Name structure 'A'.
2   Name structure 'B'.
3   Name structure 'C'.
4   Name structure 'D'.
5   Name structure 'E'.

10.17

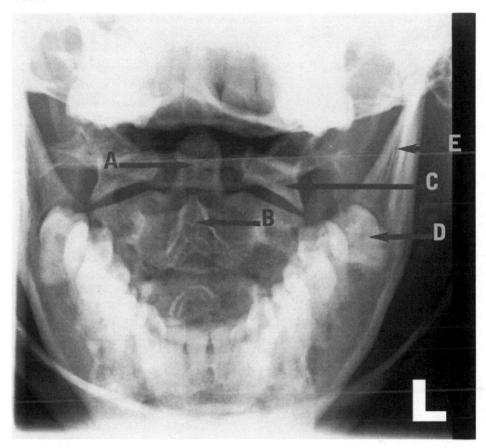

Answer the following questions.

1 Name structure 'A'.
2 Name structure 'B'.
3 Name structure 'C'.
4 Name structure 'D'.
5 Name structure 'E'.

10.18

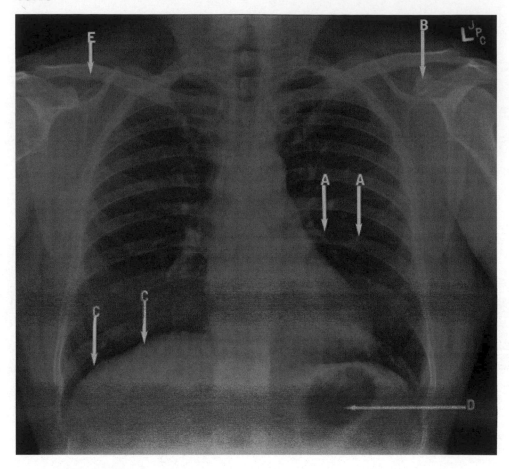

Answer the following questions.

1 Name structure 'A'.
2 Name structure 'B'.
3 Name structure 'C'.
4 Name structure 'D'.
5 Name structure 'E'.

10.19

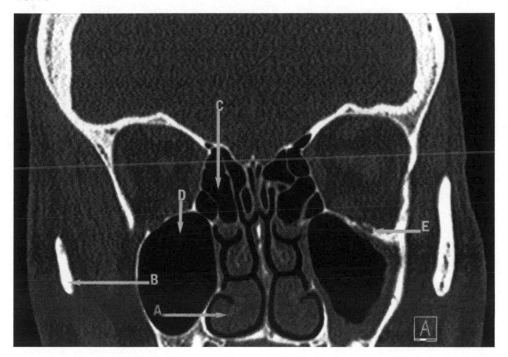

Answer the following questions.

1   **Name structure** 'A'.
2   **Name structure 'B'**.
3   Name structure 'C'.
4   Name structure 'D'.
5   Name structure 'E'.

10.20

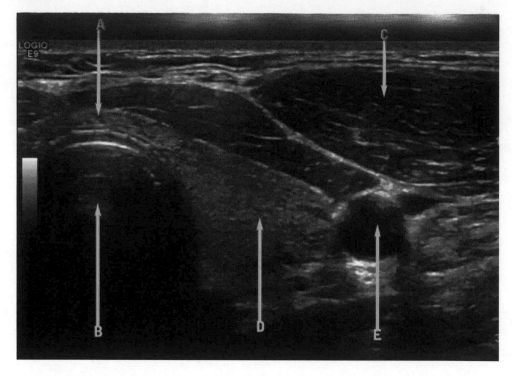

Answer the following questions.

1   Name structure 'A'.
2   Name structure 'B'.
3   Name structure 'C'.
4   Name structure 'D'.
5   Name structure 'E'.

Answers

10.1
1. Papillary Muscles Left Ventricle.
2. Brachiocephalic Trunk (Inominate Artery).
3. Superior Vena Cava.
4. Portal Vein.
5. Right Brachiocephalic Vein.

Coronal T2W MRI thorax.

The papillary muscles are attached to the mitral and tricuspid valves via the chordate tendineae. Their action is to prevent regurgitation of blood into the atria during ventricular contraction.

10.2
1. Right Internal Oblique Muscle.
2. Gall Bladder.
3. Linea Alba.
4. Body of Pancreas.
5. Retroaortic Left Renal Vein.

Axial CT Abdomen.

A retroaortic left renal vein is found in approximately 4% of patients. It is an important finding to mention in reports as it may be at risk in retroperitoneal surgery, especially during cross clamping of the aorta in vascular surgery.

10.3
1. Right Mastoid Process.
2. Left Subclavian Artery.
3. Right Internal Jugular Vein.
4. Left Vertebral Artery.
5. Right Transverse Process of C6.

Coronal CTA reformat.

10.4
1. Radial Tuberosity.
2. 1st Metacarpal.
3. Ulnar Styloid.
4. Distal Pole of Scaphoid.
5. Olecranon.

Lateral forearm radiograph.

Due to the lack of a side marker, laterality cannot be ascertained. The radial tuberosity has the attachment of the biceps brachii on its rough posterior surface. Anteriorly it is covered with a bursa between the tendon and bone. Biceps brachii is a powerful supinator of the forearm and also assists brachioradialis in elbow flexion.

10.5
1   Parotid (Stensen's) Duct.
2   Secondary Parotid ductules.
3   Body of C3.
4   Hyoid Bone.
5   Opposite the 2nd upper molar.

Parotid Sialogram.

10.6
1   Right Fabella.
2   Right Patella.
3   Right Fibular Head.
4   Right Tibial Tuberosity.
5   Right Patellar Tendon (more correctly Patellar Ligament).

Horizontal beam lateral (HBL) radiograph right knee.

The fabella is a sesamoid bone found in the lateral head of gastrocnemius in up to 30% of individuals. The Latin name means 'little bean'. It is important as it may be mistaken for a loose body, fracture fragment or osteophyte.

10.7
1   **Right Ischial Spine**.
2   Right Iliac Crest.
3   Left Sacroiliac Joint.
4   Right Transverse process of L2.
5   Descending Colon.

AP abdominal Radiograph.

10.8
1   Frontal Sinus.
2   Body of Right Zygoma.
3   Frontal Process of Right Zygoma.
4   Right angle of Mandible.
5   Left Coronoid Process of Mandible.

Occipitomental radiograph.

10.9
1   Distal Phalanx of Right Index Finger.
2   Right 5th Metacarpal.
3   Right Lunate.

4   Right Radial Styloid.
5   Radial Side Scaphoid Tubercle and Trapezium, Ulnar side: Pisiform and Hook of Hamate.

Dorsopalmar radiograph of right wrist.

Many mnemonics exist to aid recall of the carpal bones. One of the most popular (and tame!) is: Some Lovers Try Positions That They Can't Handle.

Proximal row: Scaphoid, Lunate, Triquetrial, Pisiform.

Distal Row: Trapezium, Trapezoid, Capitate, Hamate

10.10
1   Right Femoral Artery.
2   Right Ligament of Head of Femur (Ligamentum Teres).
3   Right Gluteus Maximus.
4   Left Femoral Head.
5   Bladder.

Axial T1W MRI femoral heads.

10.11
1   Greater Tuberosity of Left Humerus.
2   Left Glenoid.
3   Anatomical Neck of Left Humerus.
4   Left Radial Head.
5   Left Coronoid Fossa.

AP radiograph left humerus.

The anatomical neck of the humerus is a groove separating the head from the tubercles. It is the line of attachment for the joint capsule. The surgical neck lies more obliquely below the tubercles and represents the most common site of proximal humeral fracture.

10.12
1   Conus Medullaris.
2   Body of T10.
3   Nucleus Pulposus of L2/3 Disc.
4   Spinous Process of L2.
5   Cauda Equina.

Sagittal T2W MRI lumbar spine.

The conus represents the most distal part of the spinal cord. It is found at the level of L1/2 in most adults. Distal to this a bundle of nerve roots continue as the cauda equina (Latin: 'horse's tail').

10.13
1   **Right Obturator** Foramen.
2   **Shaft of Right** Femur.
3   Right Sacroiliac Joint.
4   Right Lesser Trochanter.
5   The Common Tendon of Psoas Major and Iliacus (Iliopsoas).

Oblique lateral radiograph right hip.

10.14
1   Spinous Process of C2.
2   Epiglottis.
3   Thyroid Cartilage.
4   Occiput.
5   Trachea.

Lateral cervical spine radiograph.

10.15
1   Falx Cerebri.
2   Cisterna Magna.
3   4th Ventricle.
4   Quadrigeminal Cistern.
5   Trigone of Left Lateral Ventricle.

Coronal T2W MRI brain.

A cistern is a subarachnoid space filled with CSF. The cistern magna is the largest and lies between the cerebellum and the medulla oblongata. The quadrigeminal cistern lies between the splenium of the corpus callosum and the cerebellum. It contains the great cerebral vein (of Galen).

10.16
1   Right Transversus Abdominis Muscle (Tranversalis muscle).
2   D2.
3   Inferior Vena Cava.
4   Jejunum.
5   Left Common Iliac Artery.

Coronal T2W MRI.

The fluid filled stomach and duodenum are clearly seen on this T2W study.

10.17
1   Dens of C2.
2   Spinous Process of C2.
3   Left Lateral Mass of C1.
4   Left Lower 3rd Molar.
5   Left Ramus of Mandible.

OPG.

10.18
1 Left 8th Rib.
2 Left Coracoid Process.
3 Right Hemidiaphragm.
4 Gas in Fundus of Stomach.
5 Right Clavicle.

PA chest radiograph.

10.19
1 Right Inferior Concha.
2 Right Ramus of Mandible.
3 Right Ethmoidal Air Cells.
4 Right Maxillary Sinus.
5 Left Infra Orbital Canal.

Coronal CT facial bones.

10.20
1 Isthmus of Thyroid Gland.
2 Trachea.
3 Left Sternocleidomastoid Muscle.
4 Left Lobe of Thyroid.
5 Left Common Carotid Artery.

Axial USS thyroid gland.

The internal jugular vein can be seen lateral to the common carotid artery. It is distinguished from the artery on scanning as it is easily compressible under the USS probe.